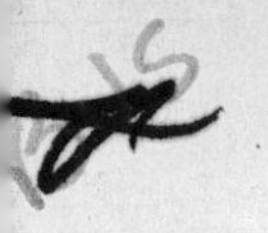

Computers and your health

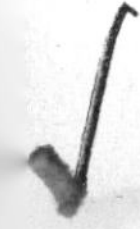

COMPUTERS AND YOUR HEALTH

The Essential Manual for Every Computer User

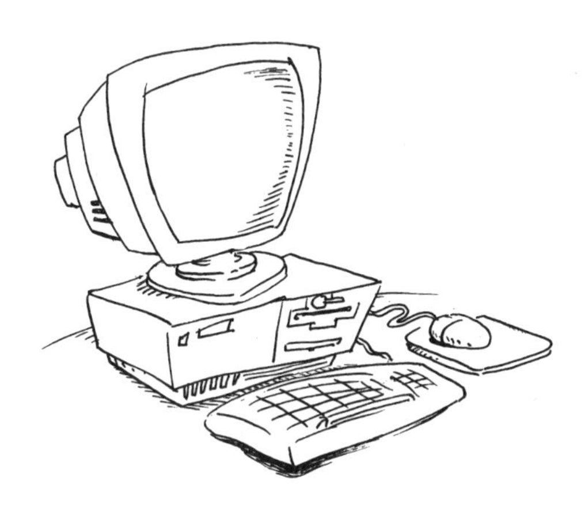

JOANNA BAWA

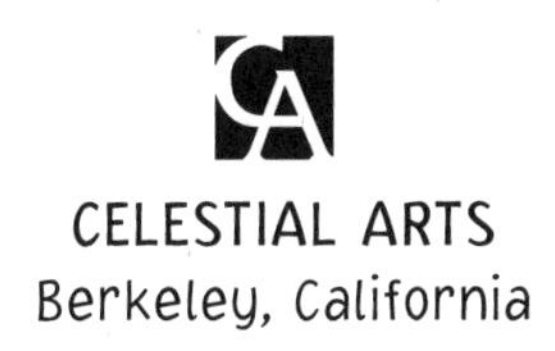

CELESTIAL ARTS
Berkeley, California

To Karan, with Love

Celestial Arts
P.O. Box 7123
Berkeley, California 94707

Library of Congress Cataloging-in-Publication Data
Bawa, Joanna.
Computers and your health: from eyestrain to wrist pain/by Joanna Bawa.
p. cm.
Includes bibliographical references and index.
ISBN 0-89087-809-9
1. Video display terminals—Health aspects. 2. Computers—Health aspects. I. Title.
RC965.V53B39 1996
613.6'2—dc20 96-21051
CIP

A Kirsty Melville Book

Cover design by Toni Tajima
Text design by Catherine Jacobes
Illustrations copyright © 1996 by David Uttal

Printed in the United States
First Printing, 1996

1 2 3 4 5 / 00 99 98 97 96

Contents

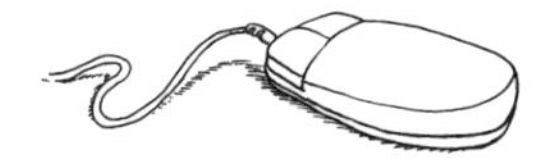

Acknowledgments

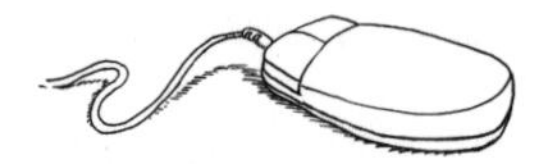

GRATEFUL THANKS ARE EXTENDED to the following people, whose generosity, patience, expertise and time were invaluable in the writing of this book:

Dr. Stephen Pheasant, consulting ergonomist; Rupert Goodwins, writer, technologist, video game reviewer with *The Independent*; Edgar Wilson, physical therapist; Dr. Kim Burton, osteopath, Huddersfield; Dr. David Thomson, optometrist, City University; Richard Teverson, technical consultant, Philips Consumer Electronics; Alan Cuthbertson, technical consultant, Philips Consumer Electronics; Sheila Lee, osteopath and clinical ergonomist; Jim Birch, Key Tronic Corporation; Anthony Steven, Healthware, York.

Preface

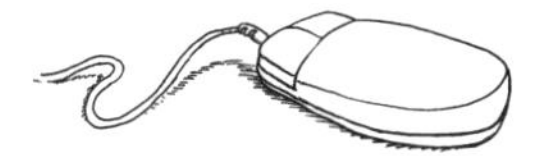

IN THE PAST TEN YEARS ALONE, the computer industry has contributed to the biggest technological revolution of the twentieth century and has changed the way we live, work, and interact with the world around us in many dramatic ways. How it contributes, and in what areas, is not always so clear.

In terms of volume and accuracy of work, computers have helped. We can now deal with more data in less time; we can process more accurately to reveal more meaningful information than previously. Computer power can control complex machinery and instruct it to perform tasks well beyond the capabilities of its operations; it can achieve more and greater goals in less time. Computers contribute to important fields like medical and scientific research and practice, and to small but vital areas such as traffic light sequencing and adding up supermarket checkout bills. They are part of our working lives and our leisure, and their role and importance seem to be increasing all the time.

One thing computers do not seem to be very good at is making us happy. Admittedly, that was never an objective: computers were only ever tools designed to serve us. But surely some element of human happiness should be the byproduct of better tools? In practice it doesn't always seem to work like that. Part of the success of the computer has been at the expense of the human employee. To add insult to injury, the gains achieved through computers last only until competing organizations acquire the same level of computer power.

Although computers stand to benefit the human race as a whole, it is people who are paying the cost. Whether or not this *should* happen is beyond the scope of this book, but it is becoming clearer that it *is* happening. From simple, measurable complaints like headaches and stiff necks, to more serious medical disorders such as eyestrain and repetitive strain injury, to complex social problems like stress, unemployment, and work alienation, people are paying the price of rapid computerization at home and at work.

This handbook attempts to identify what those human problems are and how we can deal with them in the context of a society in which computers will certainly continue to play a significant role. Although each chapter deals with separate issues, none of them can really be addressed without consideration of the others. The theme is therefore the holistic nature of our relationship with computers and holistic ways of dealing with them. In the course of my research, it has become apparent that small health problems rarely occur in isolation—a headache, for example, may be one of many minor symptoms which a person experiences during computer use. More serious health complaints tend to be accompanied by more serious occupational and relationship difficulties and, generally, hard-to-diagnose ailments often seem to be indicative of deeper discontent with work, relationships, and life in general.

Computers & Your Health is not intended to be alarmist. It does seek to identify and discuss the health problems which appear to have some relation to computer use. It also makes clear when these problems are minor complaints (such as headache), or restricted to a tiny proportion of the population (such as electrical hypersensitivity). Where more serious health issues appear to be at stake (for example, repetitive strain injury or electromagnetically-induced miscarriage), the existing research evidence is thoroughly reviewed. Invariably, it is inconclusive and tends to point to wider social factors as significant contributors in these cases.

It short, it appears that the computer in isolation is rarely to blame for the illnesses we suffer. Instead, it is the way in which computers are used, the context in which we are expected to use them, and the degree of control we have over them that determines our state of mind and body. Treating an isolated complaint will, at best, provide short-term relief. My emphasis is, therefore, largely on the *prevention* of computer-related illness rather than the *cure*. Most of the complaints discussed in this book need to be understood and treated as part of the wider issue of our whole relationship with computers, as we slowly come to terms with the new social and occupational order of which they are a part.

CHAPTER 1

Coping with Computing

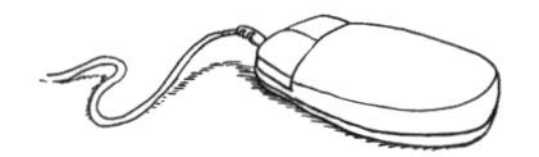

IMAGINE A TOOL THAT CAN BE ADAPTED for any purpose. It is not designed for a single task—so it can be used for *any* task. It is fast, accurate, and it doesn't get tired. It can run through immensely complicated calculations in seconds, and it won't make a mistake. In the hands of a competent programmer or designer, it can be adapted to control just about anything you care to name: factory production lines, kitchen appliances, office systems, automatic tellers, medical diagnostics, silicon chip design, picture postcard design. It is the center of one of the largest, fastest-growing, and most successful industries of the twentieth century, and it is rapidly becoming something no home can do without.

Unless you have deliberately insulated yourself against this phenomenon and taken steps to avoid all contact with the beast, you will have met a computer. They are small now, and powerful, and have become an integral part of most American jobs. Even people who don't work directly with computers are almost certainly influenced by them in some way, from the youngest school child to the most powerful executive.

How has this happened? What do computers do that makes them so indispensable? To most people and companies who invest in computer power, the answer is that computers manage the calculating and controlling functions that people used to do, only they do them faster, more efficiently, and more reliably. And once one company begins to see its profits perk up under the influence of a computer, all its competitors have to buy computers too, just to keep up.

The way it works is simple: Information is as valuable a resource to companies as capital or people—information about market trends, buying preferences, customer biographical and geographical profiles, economic reports, customer feedback, and statistical analysis. Computers and the software they run provide this information by collating, analyzing, summarizing, presenting—and even transmitting—raw data to the people who need it. Decisions are often made solely on the basis of this information: Small decisions about how many cookies to serve at meetings; internal decisions about recruitment policy and job titles; corporate decisions about future growth and marketing; life decisions about whether to launch a new business at all. Without information being accessible, relevant, and up-to-date, the chances of such decisions becoming misguided and expensive mistakes are much larger. Without the help of a computer, even good decisions will be made just too late. It works at a personal level too. Not only do computers provide information to boards of directors in multinationals, they are being used more and more in small companies, partnerships, one-person businesses, and personal finance for the same reason: More information, faster information, better information.

Hand in hand with the "information" idea is the "productivity" idea. Computers make you more productive. Because they are faster, more accurate, and more reliable, they let you get more work done in less time. Word processors have eliminated carbon paper, correction fluid, and spelling mistakes, so the first time you print a document, it will be perfect. And if it's not, it is easy enough to go back and make the amendments directly on the screen. Spreadsheets and accountancy software mean you can balance your own books and calculate your own tax returns—no need to employ an accountant, no need to make appointments with a financial adviser. That means money management is cheaper and can be done more quickly—hence, you are more productive. When you work with a computer, either in an office or at home, you get more done in less time.

Timely information and increased productivity are the promises that hardware and software manufacturers make to us when we buy their products—but that's not all. Even if we don't care about these promises, we have to pay attention because our competitors almost certainly do; so we have to get more and more involved in computers just to keep up with competing businesses, rival colleagues, even the neighbors.

Doing more in less time is a tempting idea for the hard-pressed executive, solo business manager, or busy home-worker. But does it really work like that? Are we doing more in less time? And if we are, where is all the time we are supposed to be saving—the time, computer manufacturers assure us, we will have to spend doing things we would rather do?

Ironically, the opposite seems to be happening. In the 1990s, Americans are working more hours per day than ever. A three-day working week remains as elusive as ever; all our efforts seem to be directed towards packing in more work per hour, more productive hours per day, than ever before. The development of smaller and more powerful computers has brought that urgency into our free time and our home time; we are encouraged to work in the car, on the plane, and in the living-room. If you have access to the full complement of today's computing technology—portable computers, networks, modems, telecommunications, and satellites—*you need never stop working*. You can work wherever you are and whatever time it is. There is simply no excuse to stop.

Is *this* a tempting idea? Or is it more like some sort of technological nightmare in which computers control our lives from birth until death, morning, noon, and night? The answer lies somewhere in between. Using computers, we *are* doing more in less time. But instead of stopping and saying, "I've done my day's work in two hours, so from now on I'll just work for two hours a day," we are saying, "I've done my day's work in two hours, so for the next two hours I'll do tomorrow's work, and for the two hours after that I'll do the day after's work, and by the end of the day I'll have done a week's work so that tomorrow I can start next week's work!" The people who pay us to work for them are saying the same thing. Instead of going home to relax after taking on so much extra work, we are packing up our notebook computers, loading our floppy disks, going home to our home computers and starting again in the evening. Computers can now dial in to telephone lines and talk to each other, so you can even do your research from home, dialing into databases and drawing from electronic information at any time of the day or night. We can't even snatch a few minutes during the commute to work any more: That's a precious hour when you could be using your notebook computer to type an article, design the front cover, or prepare a presentation on the benefits of desktop publishing software.

This, of course, is an extreme example of computerization. Nobody really expects anyone to work 24 hours a day and nobody could, even if they wanted to. But the point is, we *are* doing more, so we are *expected* to do even more. The whole pace of our working lives has accelerated, and the boundaries between work and home life have become more blurred. And the more this happens, the more we need it to happen. If a sales executive from a rival company gets hold of a notebook computer and the latest software and starts to analyze data about your customers, you have to get hold of the same software, or better, and analyze data about his customers. And if you do get better software, he is going to get the next, improved version. The freelance designer, previously reliant on pen and paper, begins to lose contracts to other designers who are using computer-based design software to produce better artwork in half the time. She buys her own computer and software and starts to win again, clients' expectations rise, and the design community starts shopping around for better, faster software to meet these expectations.

So it goes on. The acceleration in computer technology has triggered an acceleration in the rate at which we work, the quality of the work we can produce, and the expectations of those for whom we are working. It has also made more working hours available to us (and our competitors) than ever before, with no means of managing this time. It is an acceleration driven by computers, which will continue to increase so long as computers and software continue to increase in power, portability, sophistication, and availability. And all indications are that they are still *only just beginning.*

Why working is bad for you

As with everything that infiltrates our lives so thoroughly, there are side effects. The demand for more work, higher productivity, and longer hours is behind one of the modern epidemics of technological societies: Work-related health disorders. We are finding that the limit to the amount of work we can do is not the equipment we use, or the time we have available; it's ourselves. The human operator is now the weakest link in the automated chain; prone to tiredness, bad moods, headaches, off-days, and arguments with family members. So even though our computers are humming along, producing the words, numbers, and statistics we demand at all hours, we still need to sleep, eat, relax, and get away from work. You, our computers seem to be telling us, are holding everything up! If it wasn't for you, I could have this job done in moments! This feeling adds to the pressure we are already under; before long, this combination of stress and pressure can actually make us ill.

We have all heard about stress. It has always been around, but only very recently has it acquired formal recognition by most doctors as a modern-day disease. Since then, stress seems to have thrived and multiplied, affecting many people in many ways. Just thinking about computers is enough to induce it in some people; others suffer stress as a result of prolonged sitting in front of a computer screen without a break. On the other hand, it is probably more stressful to have no work at all if computerization removes layers of jobs. Stress is undoubtedly a factor in the epidemic of work-related health disorders which have begun to appear in the news. We are hearing more about employees whose health has been damaged, sometimes irreparably, by the work they do; increasingly, stress is cited as the primary cause.

Stress: The foundation of all illness?

Despite years in the spotlight of academic research, stress remains a poorly defined term with a wide range of antecedents and effects. *Stressors* are usually thought of as the precursors which may cause anxiety; *strain* refers to the consequences of being in a stressor-laden environment; so *stress* is often regarded as the manifestation of strain. When it gets to the point where we can feel our blood pressure rising, those worry lines getting deeper, or just plain frustration and panic, that's when we are exhibiting the *stress response*. Almost all aspects of computer-related injury involve some element of stress. This will become clear as you read through the book, so it helps to understand the nature of stress and the mechanisms by which it affects us.

What makes different people more or less vulnerable to stress? It begins with the person you are and the temperature you are born with. Our upbringing, life, experiences, and the examples of behavior we see around us, as well as our innate personality type, all influence the way we perceive and deal with difficult situations. Self-esteem and the support of people close to us affect the perception we have of our own capabilities, and the extent to which we can predict and control stress contributes to our reaction. Different people have different perceptions of the same situation. Asked to give a presentation to the board of directors, one individual will crumble in terror, overwhelmed by the responsibility and fully expecting failure and humiliation. Another may grasp the opportunity with relish, delighted at the prospect of impressing his or her superiors. Both will undergo physiological changes and exhibit a stress response to some extent. For one, the task creates anxiety which inhibits performance; for the other, the anxiety may actually enhance performance. Simple optimism can make stressful events appear less stressful, as can the ability to think about such events in a wider context. It may seem a disaster when the photocopier breaks down just as you are about to make copies of that presentation to the board. The person who can take the view that it is not so important, since copies can be provided later, will feel less stressed than the person who sees the breakdown as the last nail in the coffin of what was going to be a dreadful presentation anyway.

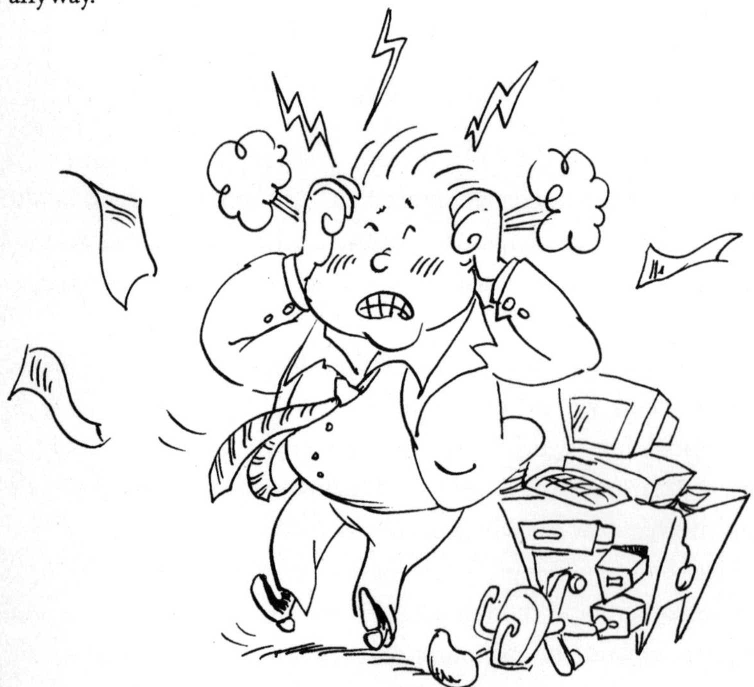

Stress in the workplace

Some people, for genetic reasons, are simply more likely than others to develop stress-related illness such as high blood pressure, although diet and exercise are of course important here, too. A diet high in sodium or being overweight can contribute to high blood pressure and the effectiveness of the way we respond to stressful events. However, careful eaters with a genetic predisposition to high blood pressure are still more likely to develop this condition than their non-predisposed colleagues. The same is true for many sufferers of stomach ulcers. Stomach ulcers are caused by the excessive secretion of digestive acids, an event which is itself triggered by stressful events. Stress doesn't have much relevance to those individuals who have naturally high levels of stomach acidity; even in a completely calm environment they can still develop stomach ulcers and, when exposed to stressful events, they are far more likely to develop ulcers because a genetic predisposition is already there.

We don't have a great deal of control over our temperament either. Researchers into heart disease have identified a series of behavioral traits which make up two extreme personality types, Type A and Type B, and which are of particular significance in stress-related illness. Type A people tend to be intensely competitive, aggressive, and determined to succeed at whatever they do. Type B personalities, on the other hand, are far more easy-going. They are more concerned with balance in their lives, and are frequently prepared to give up more money or corporate perks in return for an easy life. Type Bs rarely treat "winning" as a virtue in itself, but see value in the experience of participating and learning. They often require encouragement to complete projects and will abandon tasks that fail to engage their interest. Most of us fall somewhere between Type A and Type B, but people who exhibit most, or all, of the Type A characteristics are significantly more likely to suffer from coronary heart disease. If such people are working in an environment laden with stresses (whether computer-related or not), the chances of disease are higher still.

WHAT HAPPENS IN STRESSFUL SITUATIONS?

The human stress response is very much a leftover from our days of fighting for survival in the caves and jungles of prehistoric times. When under sudden stress, we experience drastic alterations in many of our organ systems.

If the stressor is more indirect or drawn-out (perpetual frustration, irritation, or anxiety), the effects are simply slower and more insidious. Either way, the same body systems are used to deal with stress situations. The brain begins to secrete adrenaline and noradrenaline, then we experience an acceleration in the heart rate, increased blood pressure, and sweating. Breathing becomes more rapid, which reduces the level of carbon dioxide in the blood and enriches it with oxygen. In this state, a person is poised for action, be it fright, fight, or flight. In the work situation, however, or other stressful events of modern life, none of these courses of action is generally appropriate.

When no physical action takes place, the body is left awash with a flood of chemicals it cannot use. If rapid breathing continues (hyperventilation), the acid balance of the blood changes and may cause dizziness, tingling sensations, and faints. The lack of muscle activity means other ways must be found to flush out the adrenaline and often this may take hours, rather than minutes as the body intends. The muscles, highly oxygenated and richly supplied with blood, begin to ache and tire and digestion must continue without the necessary blood transportation happening around it. If the stress response is invoked just once or twice and not used, the effects will be negligible. If it happens repeatedly, under the influence of tight deadlines or impossible workloads, for example, the sufferer becomes more and more susceptible to illness. There are direct effects: From indigestion, sleeplessness, and heart palpitations, to stomach ulcers and coronary illnesses. It is possible to say that a stressed person is more likely to develop these conditions than an unstressed person, but it is rarely possible to say *how much* more likely, or when the first symptoms will appear. The indirect effects of stress are a wide range of mental and physical disorders, including disturbed sleeping habits, irritability, and generalized anxiety as well as apparently unrelated illnesses. Repeated stress responses suppress the immune system, making us more vulnerable to everyday infections such as colds and flu, and it is possible to get into a cycle of stress, poor performance, and more stress.

STRESS AT WORK

Isolated catastrophic events—the death of a loved one, breakup of a relationship, or unexpected job loss—induce a stress response which may overwhelm a person. Work stress, however, takes time to make itself felt. Sometimes, *stress* and *work* feel as if they are words which can be used interchangeably. Mounting workloads, uncooperative colleagues, miserable pay, and long hours conspire to make even the most interesting job seem little more than a grinding task from morning to night. Much of this is beyond our control, but there do seem to be common factors underlying the experience of stress at work.

The most important two elements influencing our vulnerability to stress are *control* and *responsibility*. So long as these two components are balanced, and suit a person's ambitions and needs, it is likely that such a person will be resistant to the stress of minor irritants at work. By contrast, the most direct route to stress and related illnesses is to take a job where much is demanded and little provided to allow you to meet those demands. For example, a secretary may be promoted to junior management level and expected to shoulder additional responsibility for decision-making and managerial functions, which increases her job demands. If this is not accompanied by greater resources being made available to her, or an increase in the extent to which she can arrange her working hours or assert authority over more junior staff, the likelihood of her developing a stress-related illness increases. If her additional responsibilities include greater authority and control, she will be better equipped to cope.

The point is that where people are doing demanding jobs, they need freedom to make their own decisions about how and when responsibilities are met. Less demanding jobs don't require such freedom: Many people at this level prefer more structure to their jobs and smaller, more numerous goals to meet. If this goes too far, however, stress reasserts itself. If no decision-making or personal input is required, workers experience boredom and isolation and find it increasingly difficult to generate creative thought. They are able to contribute less and less to their working environment, since so little is required of them.

Within this broad context, our working lives are fraught with other types of stress. Being asked to do a complex new job without any form of training is stressful, as is covering for a colleague who is suddenly with no notice. Conflict with superiors or subordinates is exhausting and can sometimes lead to uncertainty about exactly what our job role is, what is required of us, and what our responsibilities are. Even the environment in which we work can be a potent source of stress, especially where we are exposed to noise, poor lighting, dirt, or extreme temperatures.

It is important to remember that no one can predict exactly how an individual will respond to stress, or even whether stressors will be perceived as such by everyone exposed to them. The response any single individual finally makes to an event is the product of a lifetime's training, molded by parental example, life experience, genetic factors, personality characteristics, and general outlook. Even if these are known, there are still many potent factors which change from day to day—marital happiness, health, financial worries, disagreements with family members or colleagues, even the weather—all of which can influence our ability to cope in a particular situation.

Computers and stress

But back to the computer. How does it contribute to the stressfulness of our fast-paced, modern working lives—if indeed it does? We have already seen how the human element is the weakest link in the chain of computerized productivity—this alone is stressful. Think how easily a piece of typing could be finished, a presentation prepared, and a column of figures added if it were not for the fact that *you* need a hot meal and a good eight hours' sleep every night. That feeling of "holding everything up" is stressful for many of us, sometimes even inducing a feeling of inadequacy. What's the excuse, after all, if that presentation doesn't get prepared on time? You can't blame your lightning-fast computer or feature-rich software—which means it must have been *you* who couldn't get it together in time.

Computers don't just go faster, though; they also control other things and make *them* go faster. Imagine a software package which just dials telephone numbers constantly. It is part of a large telesales operation, and guarantees that there will always be someone answering the ringing phone. The telesales staff don't even have to wait for the phone to ring—so many numbers are being dialed at once that there is always someone there. If more people answer a call than there are people to talk to them, the computer hangs up the extra numbers and redials them the second the previous call finishes. The telesales staff never stop talking. As one call ends, another voice is greeting them on another line; they don't have to find the number, dial it, or wait for it to be answered.

This software exists. Imagine using it—you'd have a sore throat within hours and a headache every day. Your customers wouldn't be persuaded by your bright and cheerful manner, they would be horrified by your hoarse voice, breathless speech, and panicky attempts to get them off the line so that you could go to the next caller. Whole clusters of them would be left hanging as you finally escaped to get a glass of water. Once again, the human is the weak link. In many industries, human beings are such weak links that they have been replaced altogether. The mass production of many items, from electronic components to cars, is entirely computer controlled now. Precision tasks, previously the preserve of the craftsman, are now calculated to high levels of mathematical accuracy and given to computers to manage. Whole factories can be run in the (cheap) cold and dark, since computers don't need to see what they are doing, they don't get cold, and they work all night as well.

Consider pagers and communicators, modems and portable telephones. No one likes to miss an important call, but how much do we like never to miss any call at all, no matter how trivial? All linked to electronic technology, the number of devices designed to locate us and allow us to communicate with each other is growing at a rapid rate. The idea behind the design and manufacture of pagers and mobile telephones is supposedly greater freedom. Freedom for us to be away from our desks, our homes or offices, or wherever we normally work, and still catch those important calls. But is it really freedom? Isn't part of the notion of freedom that we get away from *all* those calls—even the important ones—just occasionally, without feeling guilty? Now, if we miss a call, we don't have an excuse. If we don't get to a call or don't return one within minutes, the only reason must be that we chose not to. Forget stepping out for five minutes, forget the weekend, even forget your holiday; if you can't be contacted, you have only yourself to blame. So where's the freedom in that?

These are examples of the levels of influence and control computers are now exerting over our lives. They are reducing the discretion we have over when we are available for conversation and when we are not; when we want to work and when we want to stop. The natural breaks we rely on to stay sane are increasingly being eroded by the far-reaching power of the computer. Not only do we have less discretion, we are also experiencing a greater demand for more work. Someone is gaining a lot out of using computers, but exactly who is not always clear.

The bright side

Is there a way out of this—a way of working with computers which isn't going to cripple us or make us entirely redundant from our own lives? The answer, of course, is yes. It begins with understanding that computers are really only a tool, still very dependent on the input of their human operators in order to perform at all. When we can appreciate that the intellectual effort needed to power and direct computers is still human; and that computers are entirely meaningless without human control, human information, processing and interpretation, and human imagination, we can begin to stop feeling guilty about holding up the entire process. Computers are not making us ill, it is what we are trying to do with them and the way we are using them that can be so harmful.

With only a few years remaining, we have still got a lot to learn about living in the technological twentieth century.

CHAPTER 2

Computers: What They Do, How They Hurt, How They Help

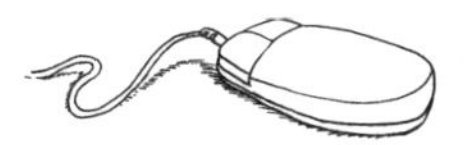

FROM A HUMAN POINT OF VIEW, the computer is exactly what it looks like—a pile of hardware—but there is obviously more to it than that, or it would not dominate our lives in the way it undoubtedly does. Since computers have given rise to such a range of health issues, it is worth trying to understand what they are really about.

The computer was a revolutionary machine when it first appeared, not simply because it could add and subtract numbers at a remarkable rate, but because *it had no specific purpose.* Prior to the invention of the Difference Engine by Charles Babbage in 1823, every piece of machinery in human possession had been created for a reason: To dig the ground, groom the horses, print letters, press carpets, light the dark. The Difference Engine was originally a specialized device for aiding in the computation of mathematical tables, and was in no sense the ancestor of the modern digital computer. It did, however, provide the inspiration for the Analytical Engine which Babbage designed in 1834, and which first raised the possibility of a machine whose mathematical power could be applied to just about anything.

That notion lies behind the proliferation of computers and software at all levels of life today, and in order to appreciate the effects and implications of computer use, at both a physical and mental level, we need to understand what goes on behind the scenes.

 Hardware

It's a common misconception to think of "the computer" as comprising three components—the system unit, the monitor, and the keyboard. In fact, there is really only one component that counts as a computer, and that is the system unit, or the plain-looking rectangular box that often acts as a sort of pedestal for the more prominent monitor. The monitor and keyboard are simply devices which allow us to enter data into the computer, and to see what comes out. Obviously, they are both essential if we are to interact with the computer in any way, but they play no part in performance, or processing of the data, and can be easily be exchanged for other keyboards or monitors. For this reason, monitors, keyboards, mice, printers, and anything that can be attached to the main body of the computer are sometimes known as peripherals.

THE SYSTEM UNIT

The system unit is the real powerhouse of the computer. It contains the power supply, the hard disk drive for permanent data storage, random access memory (RAM) chips for temporary (or working) storage, the central processing unit (CPU), the video or graphics adapter card, the floppy disk drive, a number of expansion slots for peripherals (such as printers, mice, and scanners) and points of contact for the keyboard and monitor. All of these components are connected by *bus circuitry*, a series of electronic data paths which ensure that all the components are in touch with and aware of the activities of the others.

When a computer is switched on, an electrical signal is sent to the CPU which can then begin the boot-up process. *Booting-up* is the process whereby a computer checks the functioning of all the components which are present, and loads the operating system to prepare itself for work. Despite the supreme importance to the operation of the computer, the system unit has few health implications for users. It is a relatively harmless element of human interaction with computers—far more significant are the monitor, keyboard, and peripherals. The following sections are designed to familiarize computer users with these and other components before placing them in the context of health.

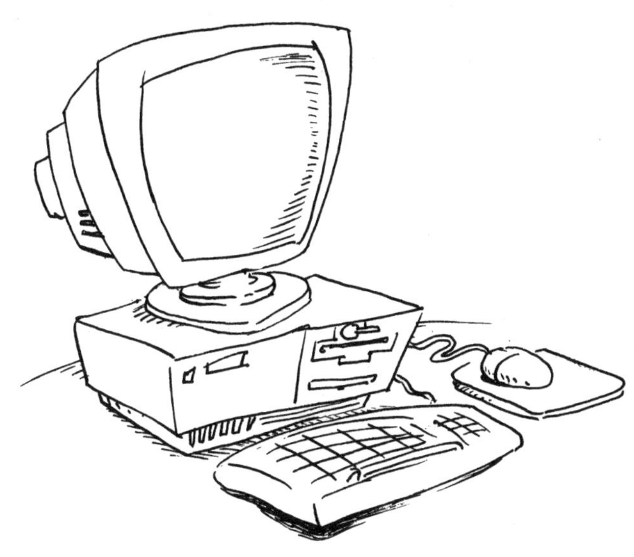

A desktop computer complete with peripherals: System unit, monitor, and keyboard.

THE MONITOR

Also known as the display, the monitor is your window into the workings of the computer. The first monitors produced images that were crude and difficult to read, and they were unable to cope with anything but the most basic images. Today, impossibly subtle color is routinely available and display images are smoother, more elaborate, and considerably more sophisticated than they were ten years ago.

Images are generated by three electron guns inside and at the back of the monitor. The quality of the image which we see on the screen depends on the screen's *resolution*—that is, the number of points on the screen which can display a color. Resolution is generally described in terms of lines and pixels. Lines are literally the number of rows on a screen which can display separate points of light; and pixels (short for "picture elements") are the points within each line—columns, if you like. A pixel is the smallest unit which can be used to build a screen image and is composed of tiny adjoining points of light. Early monitors were capable of displaying pictures composed of 200 lines high by 640 pixels wide; in comparison, the standard monitor today is capable of a resolution of 768 lines by 1,024 pixels.

Resolution is not simply a result of improved hardware, however, but relies in part on digital information from the graphics adapter card, located in the system unit. This card is most commonly known as a *variable graphics array*, or VGA card (or adapter) and can convert digital information into different voltage levels which vary the brightness of a pixel. The VGA card also controls the conversion of digital signals into three colors—red, blue, and green. The proportions and brightness of these three colors can be varied so subtly that it is possible for a standard VGA card to generate over a quarter of a million different shades (most of which are indistinguishable to the naked eye), even though only 256 of these can be held in memory at any one time. Monitors which use a super VGA card (SVGA) are able to display more colors at a higher resolution through the use of special chips and increased memory.

The shades selected by the computer are converted to signals which are then sent to three electron guns right at the back of the monitor within the *cathode ray tube* (CRT). This is a glass vacuum within the monitor and is the basic shell within which colors are generated and displayed. Each electron gun shoots out a stream of electrons, one for each of the three colors, at different intensities depending on the signals received from the adapter. The guns are aimed and controlled by a mechanism called a *magnetic deflection yoke*, which generates electromagnetic fields. These fields deflect the electrons as they stream from the guns and channel them towards different areas of the screen, creating the image which the screen will display. The deflected beams head towards the display until they strike the inside of the screen. This is coated with phosphor, which glows when struck by electrons. Three different phosphors are used for each of the red, blue, and green electron streams and the extent to which each glows depends on the intensity of the beam. The variation of electron beam intensity is what allows each pixel to display a different color—the effect of equal intensity is white light.

As the electron guns complete each line of the screen, they are switched off or "pulsed" for a tiny fraction of a second in order to refocus on the line below. This process, known as *raster scanning*, ensures that the entire screen is scanned by the electron guns, line by line, in a smooth and regular movement. Once the stream of electrons moves on to the next pixel in a line, the phosphor retains its glow for only a very brief period, after which it fades. To prevent the image from fading altogether, therefore, it is necessary to have the electron guns go back over it rapidly and repeatedly. This is achieved by the efforts of the magnetic deflection yoke, which repositions the guns back where they started at the end of each complete scan of the screen. The entire process is then repeated and the image refreshed.

THE KEYBOARD

Of all the computing components allegedly involved in damaging our health, the humble keyboard is the most directly incriminated. Our physical interactions with a computer are almost exclusively via the keyboard, the only exception being the mouse or other input device, and it is the intensive and repetitive nature of keyboard use that contributes most obviously to repetitive strain injury. This is odd because, of all the components which make up a computer, the keyboard has changed the least. With one or two radical exceptions (discussed later), design modifications have never progressed far beyond a slight change in the slope of the board, amendments to the curvature of the keys, and the location of the number pad. Typists faced with the original model would still feel at home.

Computer keyboards today are differentiated primarily by the technology which underlies their operation. Two main mechanisms exist: *capacitive* (known informally as "clicky") and *membrane* or *hard-contact*, known better as "squishy."

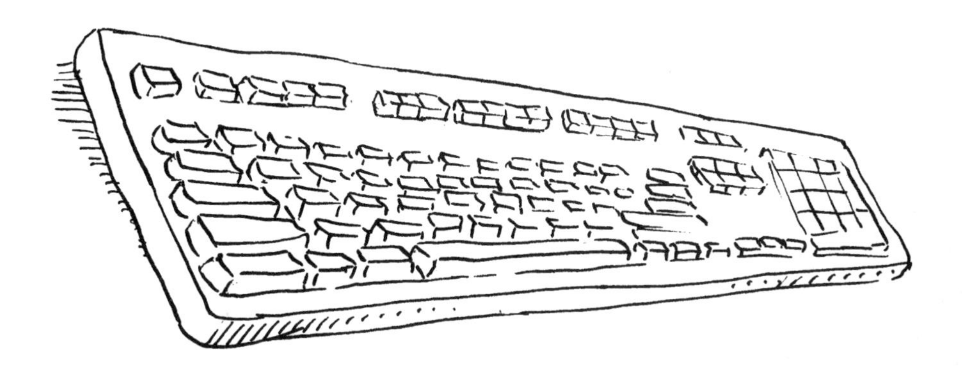

The humble keyboard: Friend or foe?

When a capacitive key is pressed, the key cap depresses a spring (which clicks) and causes a plastic or metal plunger to move towards two metallic pads of nickel, tin, and copper. The metals of the two pads are close enough to act as a *capacitor*, one maintaining a positive charge and the other a negative charge. When the plunger passes between the pads, the charge drops and creates a small current which flows directly to the circuitry of the keyboard. This charge describes the letter which is eventually displayed on the screen. When a hard-contact key is pressed, the key cap collapses a small rubber dome which in turn presses against successive layers of plastic, metal, and plastic again. The completed contact creates a charge which flows from the key to the circuitry.

The microprocessor within the computer (the CPU) constantly scans the circuitry leading to the keycaps. When it recognizes the unique code generated by each key, it immediately creates and stores a code for that key in the keyboard memory buffer. Ultimately, the stored code is translated into its corresponding American Standard Code for Information Interchange (ASCII) and can then be displayed as the correct letter on the screen.

THE MOUSE

Anything that plugs into a computer is a peripheral, but the only one (apart from the monitor and keyboard) that affects our health with any regularity is the mouse. The mouse is a product of the graphical user interface (discussed later), both elements of a concept whereby interaction with a computer became far more direct. The purpose of the mouse is to provide a more intuitive

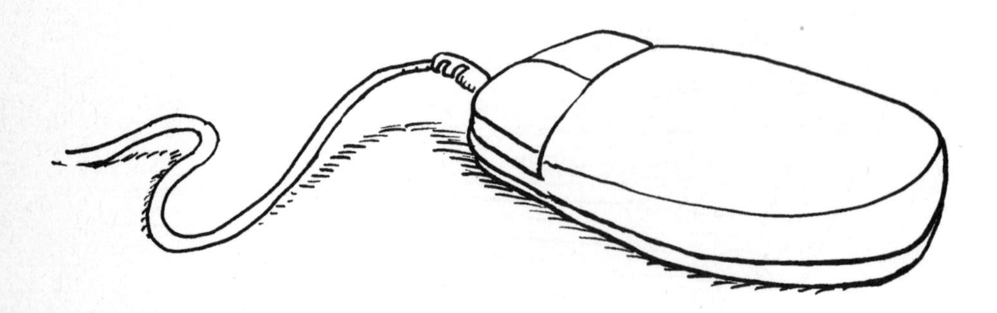

The mouse: Pointing the way to intuitive communication with your computer.

method of communicating with the computer, and to this end is sometimes called a pointing device. The idea is that hand movements made when holding the mouse are duplicated on the screen, enabling users to point to parts of the screen to activate an application (or save a file or whatever), rather than typing a keyboard command.

As a mouse is dragged across its mat (or a desk), the heavy rubber ball which protrudes from the underside rolls in the same direction. As it moves, it turns two rollers mounted at 90 degrees to one another, one of which controls horizontal and one vertical movement. If both are turned simultaneously, the effect is a diagonal movement. Movement information from the rollers is recorded by encoders which send it down the cable to the mouse software, where it appears as a corresponding cursor movement on the screen.

NOTEBOOKS

As luck would have it, the notebook computer is essentially the same in mechanical composition and structure as the full-size desktop version. The actual components that make up the system unit are small anyway, and the notebook just packs them more efficiently and reduces the amount of circuitry running between them. This can mean compromising on the amount of available disk space, but from the user's point of view, almost no functionality is lost in a notebook compared to a desktop machine with the same microprocessor. Where real savings are made is in the monitor, which obviously cannot employ the cathode ray tube technology described above. The keyboard of a notebook computer is also more compact than a full-size model, and there is a wider and more imaginative range of pointing devices available for portable use.

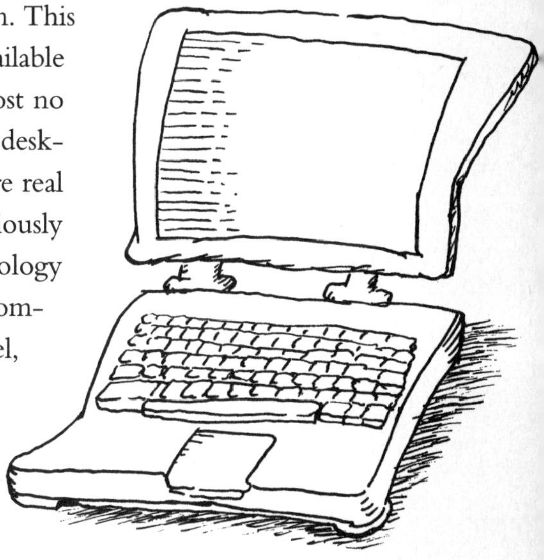

Notebook computers are the same as desktop computers, only packed more efficiently.

Notebook monitors use *liquid crystal display* (LCD) technology, which eradicates the need for the cathode ray tube and electron guns. The display begins with a fluorescent panel at the back of the screen which emits light evenly across the whole screen. The next layer of the screen is composed of liquid crystal cells which are charged or not, according to instructions received from the computer's graphic adapter. The charged cells twist to form a spiral of up to 90 degrees to their original orientation, and this forces light from the fluorescent panel to twist as well. The twisted beams pass through color filters (red, green, and blue) with a precision dependent on their orientation, and are refocused onto the final layer of the panel that we see. The proportions of each beam which get through determine the color we eventually perceive. Where the charge is applied to the cells by a few, evenly distributed electrodes, the screen is referred to as a *passive matrix screen*; where individual transistors are supplied to each cell individually, the screen is known as an *active matrix screen*. Active matrix screens generate a more precise charge and create more vivid colors, but are considerably more expensive than their passive counterparts.

The use of flat panel LCD monitors has some direct implications for the quality of the image we see, but also for our health. Monitors are most directly connected with illnesses thought to be caused by electromagnetic emissions, and these will be discussed in Chapter 4.

Software

If hardware is the heart and muscle of computing, software is the brain. At the lowest level, operating systems software controls the basic "life" of the machine—how it knows what to do when you press the ON button, how it knows to display a *k* on the monitor when you press the *k* key on the keyboard, and how it understands English commands like "copy" or "delete."

Applications software is the layer above that—what you buy on floppy disks for a specific purpose which actually enables you to perform work on your computer. It is so called because it is software you can *apply* to real tasks and objectives—you can use it to do the things you would otherwise have to do with paper, pencil, and brain. Since the spread of computers into the office, the applications software market has become one of the largest, fastest growing business areas in the entire computer industry, with application development being the mainstay of many hundreds of software companies. Its success reflects the increasing importance it has to the commercial world—and now, increasingly, the home market.

Applications software is the most diverse area of computing. The point, after all, is to apply computers to as many areas of our lives as possible. To this end, teams of developers are employed to translate human tasks and functions into applications software, the first and best known example being the transformation of typing into word processing. Today, an application (also sometimes called a "package") probably exists for every office task you can imagine: All forms of money management; graphical and artistic tasks; writing, drawing, planning, managing, arranging meetings, and sending memos. There are applications for use by specialists in areas entirely unrelated to computing—medicine, law, agriculture, or forestry, for example—where the computer is truly a tool. Increasingly, software is being applied to the home, with packages controlling personal money management at the fore, not to mention the ubiquitous games software. Because it is what we see on the screen, applications software is our most direct point of interaction with computers. It is also potentially the most difficult and frustrating aspect of human-computer relationships, and the most immediately implicated in stress, computer phobia, and general disillusionment with the whole idea.

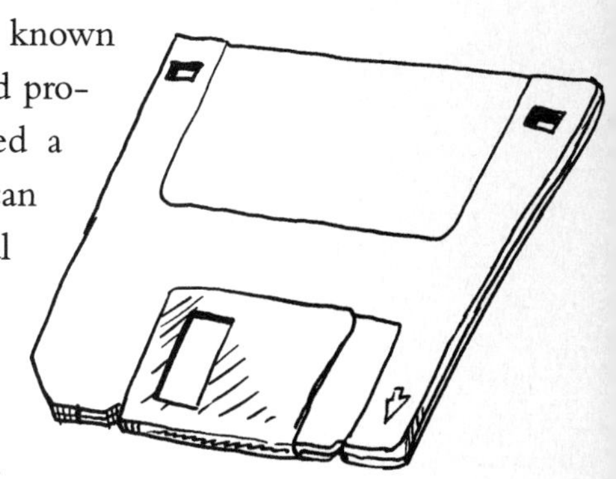

The floppy disk, a magnetic medium for storing files.

The following is a brief overview of the main categories of software. It is far from comprehensive, but describes the most widely used and successful applications in use today.

WORD PROCESSORS

The oldest and most mature application, word processing software translates clunky manual typing into a smooth electronic process. Instead of typing onto paper, word processor users type into the computer, where their work is stored electronically for later retrieval. Word processing software has become so synonymous with computers that many users regard the two as indistinguishable. Instead of switching on their computer to carry out some word processing, some people talk about "switching on the word processor." Computers, of course, are not word processors—they are the machines that run word processing software, even if they run nothing else. Well-known examples of word processing software are Microsoft Word (in all its versions), WordPerfect from Corel Corporation; and Lotus WordPro from IBM.

SPREADSHEETS

Despite being among the best-selling types of software, spreadsheets remain a relatively specialized application. Imagine the squared graph paper on which you did math at school—that's what spreadsheets often look like on the screen. They are essentially numerical, designed to take the grind out of adding, subtracting, dividing, and multiplying columns of figures. Today they do a lot more than that: Statistical functions, accounting, and advanced mathematics, all illustrated by pie charts, bar charts, and graphs. Spreadsheets are widely used by mathematicians and accountants, but they are also popular for tracking expense claims, money flows for small companies, and even names and addresses. The best known spreadsheets today are Microsoft Excel and Lotus 1-2-3.

DATABASES

As the name implies, databases are bases for storing data. One of the most useful features of the computer is its ability to store or "remember" huge amounts of data in a relatively indestructible electronic format. Databases make full use of this ability by enabling users to store information, such as names and addresses, in a way that is easily accessible. The data can be found easily by specifying a single key word for the program to look for, and many databases include a "query" facility. This lets you ask quite complicated questions, such as: "Find me all the employees in this database who live in Dallas, have worked for the company for less than a year, and earn more than $30,000 a year." Some of the most popular databases around today are Approach and Microsoft Access.

E-MAIL

"Computers" and "communication" are words frequently found together, and electronic mail (e-mail) has made the best of the available technology for this purpose. Running over a network, e-mail software provides a sort of electronic post office for a group of users who need to communicate. Messages can be typed directly at your own computer and sent across the network to other users—usually they arrive within seconds rather than days. Some offer a "chat" facility, whereby the words you type on your computer appear simultaneously on the screen of your correspondent. Well-known e-mail software packages include Lotus cc:Mail, Exchange from Microsoft, Lotus Notes from IBM, and GroupWise from Novell.

DESKTOP PUBLISHING

One of the most successful home-use applications, desktop publishing (DTP) software brings a whole range of tasks into a single product. The output of DTP software is most frequently small (or even quite sophisticated) newsletters, combining text, pictures, and publishing tricks (columns, typesetting, and elaborate design, for example). DTP was once restricted to real publishers and layout artists, but it is now so sophisticated that it is used far more widely by many different types of people who want a little more than a plain document. Most famous are Adobe PageMaker, Ventura Publisher, and Quark Xpress.

PRESENTATION SOFTWARE

Presentation software allows you to create presentations—simple as that. It is geared towards business users who need to persuade, communicate, or inform using something more sophisticated than paper-based notes or an overhead projector. Most presentation software lets you add text, graphics, and charts into each slide, and many include slides with themes or backgrounds to give a professional look. The best-selling presentation packages today are Harvard Graphics from Software Publishing Corporation and Lotus Freelance Graphics.

INTEGRATED PACKAGES

If all of the above is too much, you can buy integrated software which blends the most popular elements of applications software into a single (cheaper) product. Typically, this includes a word processor, a spreadsheet, a database, and some graphical element, although some varieties place the emphasis more on one type than another. The modules of integrated software are often scaled-down versions of the original, so the price reflects fewer features and less power. What you get in return, manufacturers claim, is better integration: Spreadsheets which can work with the information in your database; or word processors which can display the charts you prepare in a spreadsheet. Integrated software can often be the ideal compromise for a limited budget, with the best-selling products being Microsoft Works and Lotus Works.

PERSONAL MONEY MANAGEMENT

Accountancy software is generally complex and used only by accountants. Personal money management software is a new class of product, geared to the individual. It is a kind of home bank manager which keeps track of personal expenditure, income, deductions, standing orders, and direct debits—so long as you remember to tell it when these events occur! It is most popular with people who have a household budget to run, or who work from home (freelance writers and designers, for example), but some small companies and one-person consultancies can make use of this type of software too. Best known money managers are Microsoft Money and Quicken, from Intuit.

SPECIALIZED/TAILOR-MADE/TURN-KEY/ BESPOKE SOFTWARE

All these items refer to software which is designed for a specific client for a specific reason. Typically, software is specially commissioned because a client has a very specialized requirement (tropical fish husbandry planner, for example) or simply requires a larger and more complex system than can be bought ready made. Multinational corporations are frequent customers of bespoke designers, simply because available packages are unsuitable—either too small, or unable to address both the specific and general needs of the organization equally effectively.

The software design process

How does software come about? In the early days of application development, just a good idea and a clever programmer were often enough to launch a software package that could support a whole company for years. The best example of such success is possibly WordPerfect, which began life as a way of jotting down notes and has grown into one of the industry's most successful word processors ever.

Now, under the influence of commercial pressure and explosive growth in the software design market, a good idea is rarely enough to guarantee success. Software designers, like almost all commercial manufacturers, must identify a clear need for their idea before they can justify the investment in development. This involves the same process that any idea goes through: Market research, planning, designing, and testing, in order to establish its commercial worth. The product categories described above are good examples of software which fills a specific need and continues to enable its users to benefit.

The software design process is a complex and fascinating area: The following outline of the different stages provides some insight into the mysteries of the final product.

IDEA

A new software application, whether it is bespoke (tailor-made) or designed for sale as a complete package, starts with an idea. This may come from a programmer trying to apply a new design technique; from a market researcher studying the results of a survey; from a consultant or system designer asked to study people's working patterns and information flows; from a business analyst dedicated to identifying software development opportunities; and, occasionally, from a team of "users"—an unimaginative term that has come to refer to anyone who uses a computer. (You may be many things, but once you start interacting with a computer, you become a user.)

TERMS OF REFERENCE

The idea looks good. It is time to pin it down and define exactly what the proposed application is going to do (and, equally importantly, what it is not going to do). This can be a messy and prolonged process involving extensive questioning and analysis of everyone who might want to use it. Who *really* uses spreadsheet software? How important is the statistical element? Are accountants a big enough user group to justify the inclusion of a taxation module? And so on. Defining the terms of reference is really sketching out the skeleton of an application. At this stage, it also means identifying the resources such a development effort will absorb, who will provide them, and how long it will take.

BUSINESS/FEASIBILITY STUDY

An important commercial aspect of the design process, the feasibility study seeks to find out if the whole idea is really viable. With a good pen-and-pencil sketch of what the application will do and for whom, business analysts are able to test the water to see what the interest really is—in effect, what the real costs and benefits of the applications are and who would be prepared to pay for the finished product.

FUNCTIONAL SYSTEMS DESIGN (FSD)

The first stage of software design is purely functional. Designers identify the problems their product will address and then describe exactly how the application will solve the problem, often using charts to describe information flows. This stage provides a broad idea of a user's priorities and the sequences of stages or modules he or she might like to see in the finished application.

COMPUTER SYSTEM DESIGN (CSD)

The maturing FSD becomes a more precise application design, which moves away from conceptual information flows toward detailed software processes. It is still largely paper-based but concentrates on the specific operation of the software, its data, functions, development, and features. This stage also the first consideration of the interface—the part you actually see on the screen. Forward-thinking developers also include the first stages of usability testing at this stage.

SYSTEM BUILD

Once the CSD is approved by the relevant parties, the programmers can begin their job—converting the English language instructions of the designers into machine code. Depending on the size and scope of the application, programmers may work individually or in teams, each team concentrating on a specific module of the application.

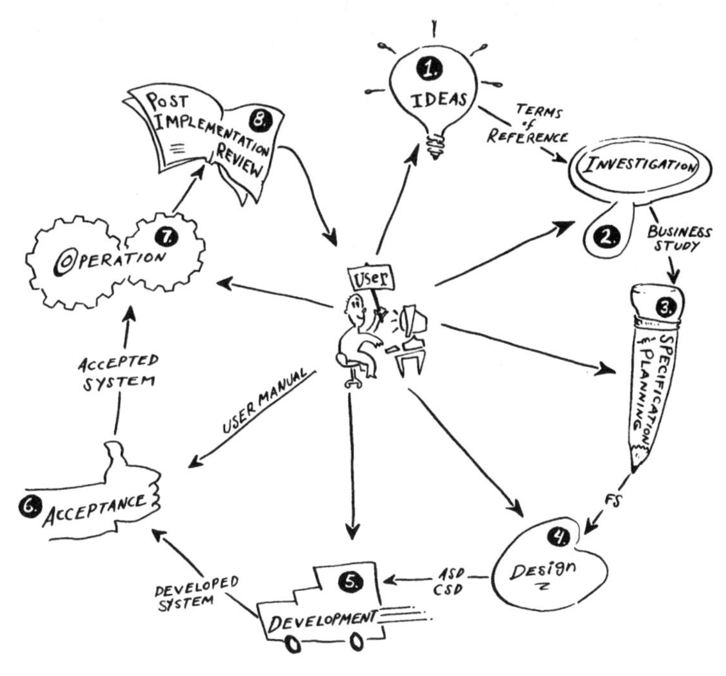

The birth (and rebirth) of a new software program.

TEST PHASE

As the modules emerge from the programmers, testing can begin in earnest. Single lines of code are tested to ensure that what goes in (the user's input) is correctly processed and comes out as expected. As each line passes the tests, it becomes part of a larger module which is tested in the same way, until eventually the modules are all merged into the final application. Testing continues at all levels, until finally the application is being tested as a single entity.

USER TRAINING AND IMPLEMENTATION

Once the application is ready to be launched on an unsuspecting world, its future users are prepared. This may mean an intensive marketing effort on behalf of the manufacturer to ensure that awareness of the product is high. For a specific client, this effort may take the form of training and the appointment of system supervisors. As the product is implemented (becomes active), its designers monitor early users closely to gauge their reactions, analyze their concerns, and begin the process of preparing the next version of the software.

POST-IMPLEMENTATION REVIEW

This stage never really stops. As users begin to explore a new application, new questions and issues arise all the time. The omission of tiny details assumes enormous proportions if they affect a frequently used or essential part of the application, and there are always new users with unforeseen needs who begin to adapt an application for slightly unexpected uses. Once the implementation is complete, it falls to the designers to monitor these changes, assess their importance, and build them into future products.

Software and sanity

What has software to do with health? Ask anyone who has ever used a poorly designed or badly presented package and you will understand. Interacting with computers (more specifically, the software running on computers) is the most daunting, frightening, and incomprehensible activity that many people can contemplate. Bad software presents a stressful paradox: You use it to achieve higher productivity, but find that it actively slows you down through its peculiar terminology, cryptic messages, and ugly appearance. Presented with such products, is it any wonder that people write off computing as a bad job? If you have a job to do, of course, you can't just give it up. It may be that you have had a product imposed on you, or a budget that allows you to contemplate only the lower range of the market. Either way, human interaction with software remains one of the most controversial areas of computing, for health reasons as well as commercial concerns.

The software interface is not a threat in the sense that repetitive strain injury is: Puzzling over the new database won't leave you crippled for life, and you are unlikely to win if you sue for high levels of annoyance. Interacting with software does influence psychological health, however and, as we will see, that is a vital factor in the development of many other illnesses. Repeated failure with a new software package damages self-esteem and reduces people's estimation and expectations of their own abilities. It is frustrating, depressing, and soon becomes boring; with nothing to show for their mental efforts, users become discouraged and may refuse to continue. Feelings of inadequacy and disillusionment may persist and spread, until reluctant computer users begin to dislike their work in general. A sense of alienation and failure casts them into a downward spiral of computer phobia and self-loathing, and productivity levels can drop below pre-computer levels. This last reason is becoming much more important, as ever-increasing numbers of people are now expected to use computers as a part of their everyday tasks, whether or not they have any interest or desire to do so. Perhaps more importantly, incomprehensible software locks people into old, slow habits of working, which effectively wastes all the time and investment that goes into a new application. Software design is a people issue as well as a money issue, and somewhere along the line these two elements are undoubtedly related.

Human-computer interaction: A growing field of study

Human-computer interaction (HCI) is one of the most actively growing fields of computing and software knowledge. It is an interdisciplinary area, drawing on the skills of psychologists, computer scientists, graphic artists, linguistics experts, ergonomists, and philosophers, and it seeks to understand just how and why so much software is so difficult to use. Researchers in HCI study good software design and what makes it good, and a vast range of complex issues related to design techniques. The justification for HCI is simple: In too many instances, computers, by forcing users to learn their languages, exert power over people. In other words, people must adapt to computers, resulting in unnatural, unhealthy, and unproductive learning and interaction.

HCI researchers believe that computers should adapt to people, and they use the techniques of experimental psychology to gather objective data about the design of software. A study of this nature might try to find the best design for a computer keyboard or monitor, or look at how colors could be used more effectively; the purpose being to determine the causes of mistakes, fatigue, injury, or plain inefficiency.

Research can be more subtle: One program, conducted by IBM, studied nine experienced users of Lotus 1-2-3 while they created and debugged three types of spreadsheets. At least one human error occurred per spreadsheet, depending on how the results were counted. Most of the errors were formula errors, a few were typographical, and one involved a mistake in rounding up or down. While the IBM experiment did not provide enough information to create a complete model about how people use spreadsheets, it did reveal that people are most likely to make mistakes when creating and modifying spreadsheets. On the basis of this work, HCI researchers were able to propose that attention to the design of certain areas of the software could reduce the most common human errors.

As an academic discipline, human-computer interaction embraces models of human thought, decision-making, and problem-solving; human information processing; the development of conceptual though; artificial intelligence; natural language processing and voice recognition. As an applied science, it seeks

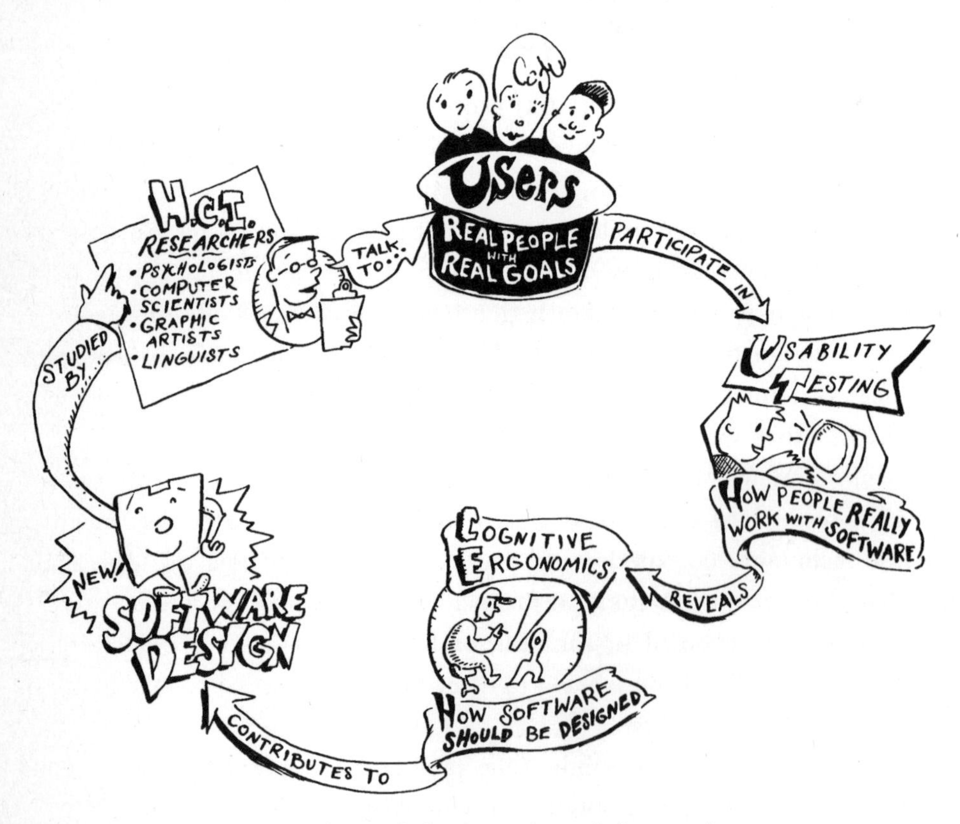

How software design is continuously improved.

to build human mental processes into software in a way that builds understanding and enthusiasm in users. HCI is obviously geared to *interaction*, and takes as its central area of concern the *interface*. The interface is broadly described as the parts of a system with which the user comes into contact physically (through touch), perceptually (via the eyes and ears), or cognitively (through the thought processes and mental activity).

The principles of sane software are not just lucky guesses, they are the result of extensive and detailed research into the way people interact with software, the concepts they acquire, the way they learn, and the objectives they have. Human-computer interaction deals with all the issues this encompasses, and uses its understanding of cognitive ergonomics to create software that possesses the property of usability.

COGNITIVE ERGONOMICS

This elaborate term describes the way our thought processes are applied to the design of a software interface. *Cognitive science* refers to the study of our mental activity: Thinking, learning, understanding, remembering, problem-solving, reasoning, and creating. *Ergonomics* is the study of people within their working environment. It traditionally places a particular emphasis on the physical environment—chairs, tables, lighting, temperature, and so forth, and the way in which these elements should be designed or controlled best to accommodate their human users. *Cognitive ergonomics* is therefore a specialized branch of ergonomics (or cognitive science, depending on your point of view) which draws on the strengths of both to achieve the optimum design for those elements of the working environment which interact with our mental rather than our physical selves.

Despite occasional appearances to the contrary, the thinking, learning, problem-solving, and reasoning power of the human user is immeasurably greater than that of a computer. Workers in cognitive ergonomics try to identify what those processes are and translate them into a software interface, the aim being to recreate our thought processes (or the *appearance* of our thought processes) within the workings of an application. This had led to the emergence of notions such as the graphical user interface and the desktop metaphor.

USABILITY LABS

It is arguable that the purpose of all HCI research and cognitive ergonomics is *usability*—in effect, the ability of software to be used (successfully). Usability labs deal with this on a very practical level, actually hiring people to interact with software while usability researchers study the difficulties they encounter and the solutions they find (if any). Most usability labs belong to university departments where research is undertaken from a very academic standpoint, although an increasing number of software manufacturers now support their own usability labs. In commercial labs, teams of volunteer evaluators are selected according to a strict profile—essentially that of the *target market*, or the sector of the population for whom the package is being built. These people participate in test interactions with the software under investigation, often trying to achieve a range of objectives which would normally be part of such use. At a micro level, usability testers might be asked to perform *drag and copy* operations, selecting items on the screen with a mouse and moving them to a different area. At a macro level, they might be asked to create a newsletter using a new desktop publishing package.

The usability lab itself is usually a simulated office with an adjoining observation room, from which researchers can watch the evaluators at work. The lab and observation room are separated with one-way glass, allowing the researchers to watch the evaluators while the evaluators see only a mirror. Although this sounds intimidating, it is designed to remove the presence of the researchers from the minds of the evaluators. Often, evaluators are filmed with video cameras so that the minute details of their interactions can be studied later by researchers. Cameras may be trained on the evaluators' faces to reveal their expressions of horror or (occasionally) delight; on their hands to track their use of shortcut or backspace keys, for example; and on the screen, to show the sequence of screen events they generate as they progress through the tasks. An essential part of usability testing is talking to the evaluators afterwards, sometimes as they watch the recordings of themselves, to identify the thought processes that led them to a particular problem or solution.

The analysis of this data is a lengthy and time-consuming process, but it reveals rich and fascinating information about the process of human-computer interaction. Principally, it identifies very specific areas of difficulty with an application, allowing the usability team to recommend changes and improvements. These can be fed back to software development teams who build them into subsequent versions of the application. Usability data can also identify far larger areas of interest—why a particular problem is always a problem for most people; why an easy task is always easy; what thought processes are most commonly used to achieve a particular goal; how we apply the knowledge about the world that we already have to new computer-based problems; and how that knowledge can sometimes get in the way.

So what has all this research come up with?

Why so much software is difficult to use

Cognitive ergonomists and usability lab researchers have identified several fundamental reasons for the failure of software design:

- The evolution of computer processes forced early users to turn all problems into procedures expressed as a sequence of logical instructions. These programs were originally intended to serve disciplines such as mathematics and engineering and do not adapt easily to non-numerical areas.
- A lack of correspondence between natural language and computer programming languages, forcing programmers to develop thinking styles radically different from those of non-programmers. This created a two-way barrier which prevented either group from satisfactorily communicating its needs to the other.
- The emergence of "expert" status for system administrators and programmers, which further removed them from the needs of "ordinary" users.
- The dominance of certain personality and intellectual types in software design, eliminating the necessary input of a wider range of thinking styles.
- The perception by many people that computing is a mystic art they cannot understand, which is best left to scientists and computer specialists.

- The inability of expert designers and users to understand the problems and concerns of non-expert (or naive) users; and inability of non-experts to express their needs in a way that experts can readily understand.
- The perception by some programmers that "mastering" the computer is a task to be met with relish, compared to the perception of users that computers are irritating or threatening machines which hinder more than they help.
- Poorly researched and implemented applications, which owe their existence more to the discovery of an interesting new technique than to the real needs of real users.

As a consequence of all this, over the years HCI researchers have been driven to develop clearer communication channels between user and designer. This has achieved deeper input into design from a wider range of sources and made an impact on software such that interface design has now become a discipline in its own right. In the hands of such specialized designers, the purpose of the interface is now primarily to conceal the workings of the software from the user, in the way that a neat dashboard and polished metal exterior conceal the workings of a car. Rather than assuming users will enjoy trying to beat the computer at its own game, HCI has enabled interface designers to show that users just want a cooperative tool that will let them get on with the job—without going mad.

Usability: Basic rules for sane software

If people are asked what they really want when they are choosing an application, they rarely say, "Something with at least three hundred and seventeen features that lets me have twelve files open at once and offers me two hundred and fifty-six colors on the screen." They are far more likely to say, "Something easy—something I can understand." This is as true for people in big companies as it is for home-based users; the reasons may be slightly different, but the desired objective is the same: People want software that will work with them to achieve a specific goal. This goal may be higher levels of productivity in a department, it may be perceived as the best guarantee that people will actually use the software, or it may just be the need to cope alone, without fear of spending many long and frustrating hours trying to describe seemingly insurmountable software problems to the local hotline-support representative.

Listening to and understanding such remarks has contributed to the massive commercial success of manufacturers such as Microsoft and Lotus, whose applications software is very consciously designed to be easy to use. The quality which makes their products so acceptable to users has become known as "usability," a term that encapsulates all the aspirations of designers to make software that people *use*. Choosing software that will leave you with your sanity can be done. It simply requires an understanding of what to look for and an opportunity to evaluate the available products with a critical eye.

Concepts

Begin by looking for concepts in the product that match whatever it is you want to do. The concept behind a word processor may be a tool for writing short, punchy memos—but you may be a novelist seeking something that is geared to cope with large volumes of text. A business manager might begin by investigating accounts software and end up with a spreadsheet, because it fits better with the concepts he or she has to deal with at work. Some word processors are conceptually similar to desktop publishing packages, including elaborate features for handling graphics and illustration. Others share a more conceptual background with the spreadsheet, offering calculators, tables, and charts. Some offer all this and more, and a price to match. Still other products have no apparent concept behind them at all. Although they may appear to be aimed at a particular need, often the "need" turns out to be trivial or non-existent, with the package relying on one minor feature as its selling point. An example might be a product that offers a new "look" to your screen, when in fact all it does is confuse the learning you have already gone through to become familiar with the old "look." Such products are often the most confusing: With no clear concept to place them in context, they become just another way of making the user feel ignorant.

METAPHORS

At a more detailed conceptual level, metaphors provide some of the best aids for users. The term *metaphor* in the software sense refers to the use of some familiar object or concept to represent a software concept, the best known being the graphical user interface. The graphical user interface (affectionately known as GUI, pronounced "gooey") is known to millions of Mac users across the world as the Mac interface, and to PC users as Microsoft Windows(TM). These two GUIs are by no means the only metaphors for the computer interface, but they are certainly the most familiar and most widely used.

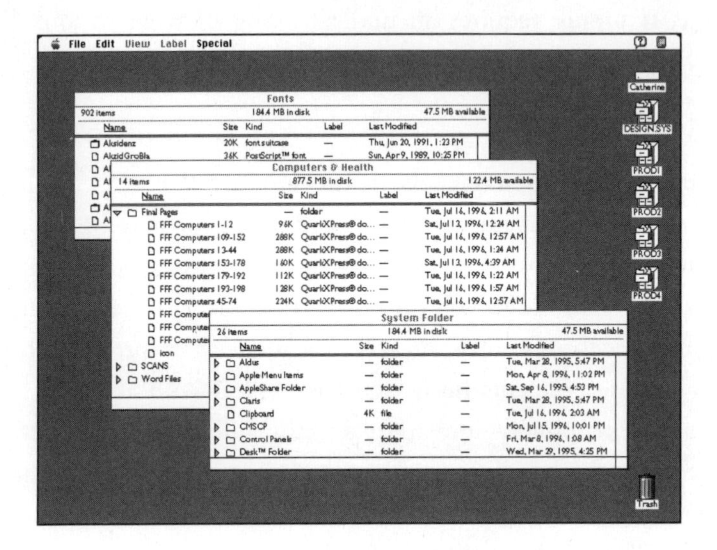

The friendly desktop metaphor.

Windows is a piece of software that provides an interface between the operating system and the user, saving you the ordeal of telling the operating system what to do directly. Windows, and other GUIs like it, conceals technical computer commands beneath visual images and words which we recognize as more familiar objects. The Windows File Manager, for example, is a small application (an "applet") within Windows which lets you create storage areas in the computer's memory and move files between them. Normally, such activities require a basic knowledge of the computer's operating system and

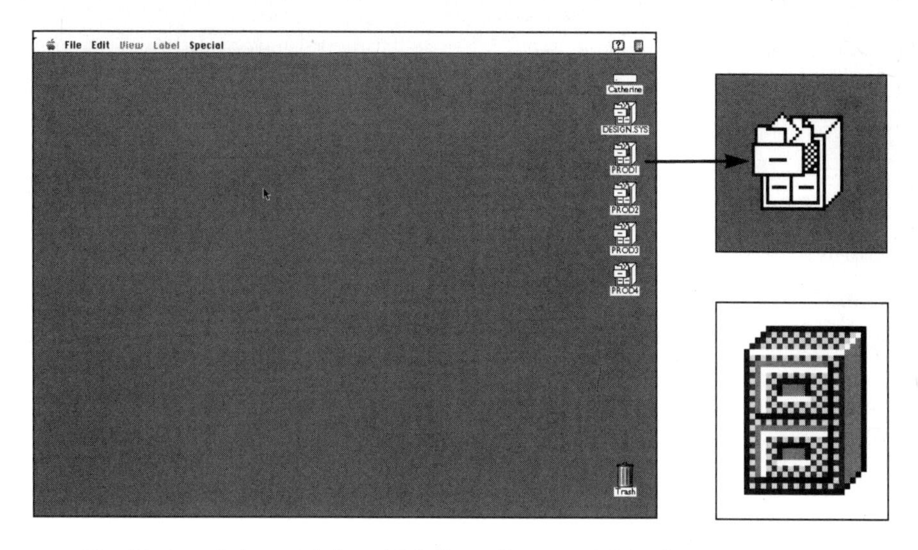

The Macintosh (top right) and Windows (bottom right) File Manager icons: Simplified computer file management.

the commands required to control it. Instead, Windows has hidden this system behind the File Manager icon, a small drawing of a filing cabinet, which converts obscure commands into intuitive pointing and dragging with a mouse. Just thinking about command languages is enough to scare some people off, but when the technical concept is hidden behind a familiar, instantly recognizable object (the metaphor) things fall into place far more quickly.

Metaphors are used most successfully when they are applied logically and consistently throughout an application. The File Manager is part of a broader "desktop metaphor" whereby the metaphor of Windows is the standard office desktop. Like a desktop, Windows displays a large, plain square area on which are held graphical "folders." Once a folder is "opened," you can see the files it has within it—Excel, maybe, or Lotus 1-2-3. Windows comes as standard with a clock, diary, and calendar; and a calculator, notepad, and card filing system. There are even one or two little executive toys to complete the desk's contents. Instead of typing obscure commands to use items on the desk, the metaphor is extended by the mouse and pointer. Simply point at the folder you are interested in, select it (pick it up) with the mouse, and open it or place it somewhere else. This metaphor works because it is based on the way we really think and work. People don't choose objects by remembering a meaningless string of characters, they choose by looking, selecting, and picking up. When this is translated into our interactions with software, we can relate to it immediately. Lotus Organizer, a diary and appointment scheduling package, has adopted the famous FiloFax as its metaphor. The graphical detail is impressive right down to the two sets of three ring binders; even the Year Planner pages "fold out" when they are selected. The yuppie accessory on which Organizer is based may be a little dated now, but the consistency with which the metaphor is used made it an instant usability success.

Once you are happy with the concepts and have grasped the metaphor of an application, it is time to look more closely at the details of the interface.

COLOR

When color displays were first developed, color was largely used on a trial and error basis, often with dazzling, headache-inducing results. The psychology of color perception now plays a far more important part in display work, and designers take the use of color much more seriously. Rather than splashing it indiscriminately on the screen, color is used to liven up an otherwise dull monochrome presentation, to reduce visual clutter but organize the display into perceptual units, or to code information. We perceive colors using special receptors on the retina of the eye, which adjust to the wavelength of the color we are viewing. Red and blue are at opposite ends of the spectrum of visible light and, when they are displayed side by side, the eye is forced to adjust to different wavelengths frequently and rapidly. It is this rapid adjustment between contrasting colors which contrasts to headache and eyestrain and is far more pronounced when the eye has to perceive colored text on a contrasting background.

Studies conducted in the early 1980s tried to determine which combinations of colors on a display were the most legible. Although most of these studies used displays with a restricted color range, they found that legibility was best determined by the lightness contrast between color combinations, and between the background and the text. Negative displays—black text on a light background—are said to be better than positive displays because of their greater overall luminance (lightness) which increases acuity and decreases the effect of glare. Some colors have a powerful influence over our emotions, with red increasing pulse rate and irritability, and pale shades of green calming us down. When choosing an application, don't be taken in by vivid and contrasting colors. Look instead for careful, subtle use of color to denote important items (incoming mail), to classify items of a similar type (names of files in a particular format), or to mark off different areas of a screen. Better still, look for applications that allow you to configure your own color scheme.

Icons

Icons are one of the central features of the GUI. Meaning "image," icons are graphical representations of tasks, functions, and features which provide an intuitive, easily recognizable label, even for those who have never used a computer before. The filing cabinet icon of Windows File Manager is an example of a concrete icon: An image of a familiar, tangible object which translates directly into a concept—filing. Others are less obvious, such as a small pig to indicate "save" or a circular arrow to indicate "repeat last action." Researchers have experimented concrete and abstract icons and found that people consistently prefer concrete images. For many actions it is simply not possible to provide a concrete image, so abstract representations have to be used (how would you represent "attach to remote terminal" graphically, for example?). The simpler and more concrete they are, the better icons are understood. Like color, they are most effective when used sparingly. Too many are dazzling and overwhelming; and, of necessity, include hard to understand abstract images. A small, but effective set of icons provides the best balance between useful tools and incomprehensible pictures.

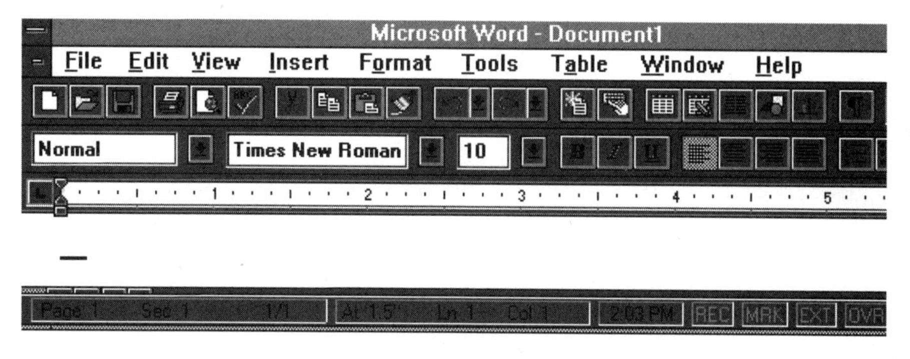

A typical toolbar, showing common icons (representations of functions).

TEXT VERSUS GRAPHICS

The GUI is essentially visual in nature (based on icons, windows, and the mouse). This makes an interface far easier to understand and more inviting to use, but beware of products which stretch graphical metaphors too far. Excessive reliance on graphics actually reduces the appeal of an interface. In the same way that icons cannot always express an abstract concept accurately, pictures, although they may be worth a thousand words, can rarely offer the precision of one. Mature software recognizes this and uses text where text is appropriate—in pull-down menus, for example, or even as a label on an icon. The nature of some applications makes a graphical interface inconvenient and sometimes almost irrelevant. Specialized, technical products are often used by experts who prefer to type directly to the operating system; people who need to work with very large volumes of data may want to minimize their computer resource overheads (GUIs require a lot of memory) to maintain speed of processing. Like color, graphics are far more effective when used carefully and thoughtfully—and avoided when inappropriate.

ERROR MESSAGES

During software use, it is not uncommon to receive error messages—usually advising the user that some procedure has been omitted, some contradictory sequence of actions requested, or a simple mistake made. The problem is that the phrasing of such error messages is often so cryptic and technical that it is impossible to decipher the nature of the problem, let alone divine a solution. Error messages designed with usability in mind have three attributes: Clear, working English; a concise explanation of the problem; and a possible solution or explanation. Often, the solution is accessed via a further button and may cross-reference topics in the on-line help or the manual. Error messages are an awkward problem for software designers, since they do not necessarily come from the application. If a user is trying to do too many things at once the computer's memory may be unable to hold them all at the same time, in which case the operating system will display a message. If the user's actions violate some principle of the interface, then the interface may display an error message, and these messages may be the ones that are misinterpreted by users and for which the application is blamed. It is worth trying to read and understand error messages and their solutions, since they are a good indication of the thought and care that lies behind the design of the overall package.

MANUALS, TUTORIALS, AND ON-LINE HELP

Nothing quite guarantees a groan the way a computer manual does. Almost universally hated by the user community, technical documentation remains one of the major headaches for applications developers: It must be included, but no one ever seems to want it. The aspect of manual use that discourages so many people is the lack of interaction. Experimental actions on the application itself (mouse clicks, hitting carriage return) invariably have some sort of feedback, and the better the application, the more likely it is that the feedback will be a constructive learning experience. Reading the manual is invariably a thankless task—dry terminology which never seems to address quite the right question, and an index which has everything in it except the one problem you have encountered. Good applications developers have approached this in a number of different ways.

First, they have tried to improve the manuals themselves. Instead of cheap, ring-bound pages of dense typing, look for professional layout and design: Well spaced text, a clear typeface, good headings and sub-headings, a well-defined overall structure and clearly marked page and topic numbers. Big applications have big manuals, so clever companies include brief Getting Started booklets or Quick Reference guides as well.

Secondly, the documentation load has been split (or duplicated) across both the manual and the on-line help, in an effort to accommodate those users who prefer to get help more directly. It is of little benefit if the on-line help is just the manual in electronic format—helpful help includes an index, a search-by-keyword facility and the same clear layout of the manual. Most importantly, it is context-sensitive—that is, it recognizes the area of the application you are working on and automatically provides help specific to that area, saving you the trouble of paging through a large electronic document.

Thirdly, developers have tried to make the user's life easier by adding electronic tutorials to applications software. Sometimes duplicated in the manual, these tutorials provide a quick overview of the purpose and capabilities of an application, along with detailed examples of common tasks. The success of these tutorials reflects the importance of conceptual understanding (discussed above), since this underlies the frame of mind in which a new user will approach an application. The closer user expectations are to what can actually be achieved, the more likely it is that the application will not be a disappointment.

Finally, efforts to make software more accessible to users have concentrated on what is actually on the screen. To make the user's interaction as immediate as possible (thus avoiding the problems of deciphering manuals, tutorials, and on-line help altogether), the interface has to be more than a series of pretty icons. Not only do the icons have to represent the functions they carry out as directly as possible through simple, concrete images, they also have to reflect the things users really want to do. A company may develop the perfect icon to represent "create an index," but if the users of that application never need to create an index, that icon will become just another piece of screen clutter. Carefully researched applications include only operations which users want on the interface. Ideally, the operations we all use all the time (open a file, save, close, help) should be the most prominent. Rarely used operations should not appear on the screen, but do need to be easily accessible if desired. Some of the more sophisticated packages include "tips" for users as they select a certain sequence of operations. For graphics packages, this may mean layout and design tips; for a spreadsheet, the tips may be geared to pointing users towards more efficient ways of performing an operation.

FLEXIBILITY AND CONFIGURABILITY

Whatever functions appear on the screen in whatever colors, and however concrete the icons are, there will always be those among the user population who have slightly different needs. In recognition of this, good applications software offers flexibility, both in the tasks it performs and in the way it looks. Where an application is aimed at novice as well as experienced users, it needs to offer the simplicity that novices require as well as the sophistication experts expect. Sometimes this means concealing advanced functions from novices, but making it clear that they are there if someone more experienced wants them. The process of removing or adding levels of functionality is called *configuration*—

it is a form of personal design which becomes more valuable as users either find themselves doing the same kind of task repeatedly, or as they gain more experience and develop preferences. Nor should flexibility apply only to the tasks available. It is important to enable users to set the color scheme; number, position, and type of icons; activity of system operations (such as autosave); and even details like the name and address of the registered user of the software. Flexibility and the ability to configure even small aspects of an application give users more control and, as we have seen, control is one of the most powerful tools for tackling and resisting stress.

Summary

It is no longer possible to interact with a computer and remain untouched by it. Carefully targeted to meet our professional (and increasingly domestic) needs, computer hardware and software have carved a vast tract for themselves in twentieth-century life and will continue to do so in the future. The health implications are wide-ranging, from the specific dangers of poor keyboard design to the wider issues of learning and understanding software, organizing the computer into our lives and discovering how to get the most out of it. As we progress, we are forced to keep pace with the rush of new concepts and applications, and the mental and emotional stress which can emerge as a side effect. In anticipation of the problems already emerging, a huge industry of designers, psychologists, engineers, and ergonomists now thrives on the health issues with which computers present us. The effort that goes into producing safe and effective computing products is enormous, but it is still one of the youngest and least organized elements of software and hardware development. Carefully researched hardware design and software usability are no longer luxuries: The technology is racing ahead of its users and it is only through the interface that we can hope to stay in the game. There is still a great deal that is poorly understood, but as we continue to think of imaginative new uses for computer power, our interactions will become more and more frequent, more prolonged, and more demanding of mind, emotion, and body.

CHAPTER 3

Repetitive Strain Injury (RSI)

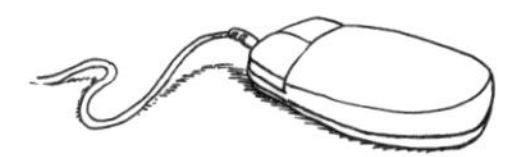

STRESS IS A RESPONSE which can be induced by the way computers are affecting the entire fabric of our work and personal lives. You don't have to use a computer to be affected by these types of change—in fact, a person may well experience stress precisely because a computer is now doing his or her job. So stress is an important health issue for non-computer users as well as computer users, although in a slightly different way. If we look more closely at computer users, stress is only one of the complaints that are turning up more frequently. Increasingly, *repetitive strain injury* is being cited as the cause of anything from slight aches and pains to serious disability and even surgery. It represents one of the most alarming health hazards to affect the computer-using population in this half of the twentieth century.

A historical account

Repetitive strain injury (RSI) is not a disease, it is the collective name for a variety of disorders affecting the neck, shoulders, and upper limbs, especially the hands and wrists. Despite coverage to the contrary, RSI has not, in fact, appeared suddenly. The reason for its sudden high profile is that it has been named—isolated as a specific condition as a result of its slowly increasing prevalence across the industrialized world. Its name explains what it is: Strain injury caused by many, many repetitions of the same action, irrespective of what that action is. The variations of RSI are known by many other commonly used names: WRULDs (work-related upper limb disorders), CDTs (cumulative trauma disorders), OCDs (occupational cervicobrachial disorders), or simple "overuse syndrome." What these conditions share is their origin in physical activity (normally in the workplace), as opposed to any viral or pathogenic origin; and the relatively specific areas they affect—the hands, wrists, elbows, shoulders, and neck.

For hundreds of years people have been working in considerably less comfortable conditions than we know today, but RSI does not seem to have been a health problem for that length of time. Yet is that really the case? The evidence suggests that RSI, and other work-related health problems, have indeed been a productivity problem for as long as people have sought work in industrial settings, but only recently have they become a human health concern.

The first documented case of RSI was recorded in 1713 by Bernardini Ramazzini, an Italian physician specializing in occupational medicine. He observed the development of "morbid affections" in workers who were required to hold "some particular posture of the limbs," or to perform "unnatural movements of the body" while they worked. He also described the daily routines of "scribes and notaries" and explained the "maladies" which resulted in terms of "first, constant sitting, secondly the incessant movement of the hand and always in the same direction, thirdly the strain on the mind from the effort not to disfigure the books by errors or cause loss to their employers when they add, subtract or do other sums in arithmetic."

In 1717, he noted of writers:

> The diseases of persons incident to this craft arise from three causes ...constant sitting...the perpetual motion of the hand in the same manner, and the attention and application of the mind...constant writing also considerably fatigues the hand and whole arm on account of the continual...tension of the muscles and tendons.

Ramazzini described one writer who, because of constant pain and weakness in his right arm, "which could be removed by no medicines," learned to write with his left hand, "which was soon thereafter seized with the same disorder."

These problems multiplied dramatically following the Industrial Revolution in Britain and America in the mid 1700s. The rise of factories and cities led to profound social changes throughout the country, especially with regard to working patterns and practices. Instead of small-scale agriculture and cottage industries, the predominant mode of employment became the factory, where conditions were harsh and brutal. Unprotected by any legislation and ignorant of health implications, factory workers toiled through long hours in cramped conditions, performing menial and often physically demanding tasks. These conditions and their effects were referred to by many social activists of the eighteenth and nineteenth centuries, particularly Charles Turner Thackruh, who wrote at length on "The Effects of the Principal Arts, Trades and Professions and of Civic States and Habits of Living on Health and Longevity" (1832). He referred generally to the harmful effects of "excess of labour," which was first documented as the symptoms of a specific illness in 1854 by Friedrich Engels. Records of neck, spine, and wrist injury were widely noted among the unfortunate employees of garment factories, and such injuries are still prevalent among modern sewing machinists. The common factor is frequent, repetitive movements of an isolated set of muscles, while the rest of the body remains frozen in the same position for hours. *Gray's Anatomy,* in 1893, spoke of "washer-woman's sprain," a swelling of the tendon caused by such movements as wringing clothes.

So RSI is not a new condition, although it has only recently become recognized and labeled as a major source of ill-health among computer users. Like the scriveners and notaries, computer users carry out small, complex movements of the hand and wrist over and over again and, inevitably, the results are the same. But unlike the workers of early industrialized life, today's employees are better able to seek redress for damage to their health as a result of computer usage.

What RSI affects

There are many elements—physical, social, and psychological—to repetitive strain injuries, which invariably have a physical manifestation. The areas affected are all complex parts of the body which work in very particular ways.

THE WRIST AND UPPER LIMB

The hand is one of the most fragile parts of our anatomy and also one of the most useful. Hands grip and manipulate, and the fingertips are among the most sensitive areas of our entire body. The hand is a very efficient group of bones, ligaments, nerves, and muscles, enabling it to perform extremely fine and complicated movement patterns. From the inside out, it consists of the carpal or wrist bones, the metacarpal bones which form the palm of the hand, and the phalanges or bones of the fingers. The joints of the hand allow for controlled movement of the bones, and the ligaments support and stabilize the bony structures. Tendons connect the muscles to the bones, and hand movement is accomplished by the intricate combination of muscles and nerves.

In its broadest sense, the hand can either be open (relaxed or extended), or closed in a powerful fist grip or a precision grip (as in holding a pen). As a gripping style becomes more precise, the fingertips are increasingly important and the muscles of the palm and wrist less so. Keyboard users work with the hand open and the fingers extended, requiring small, precision movements which are repeated over and over again. The largest and most important ligament in the hand attaches to and travels between the metacarpal heads along the entire width of the hand, where it provides support and stability. Full extensibility of this ligament is necessary for grasping and prehensile activities. If its mobility is restricted because of traumatic scarring or overuse, for example, function is greatly hampered. The ligaments of all finger and thumb joints provide important joint stability.

Nearly all the tendons of the hand pass through the carpal tunnel, along with the median nerve which provides sensation to the hand, branching into motor and sensory nerve fibers. It is the extensor tendons which are most likely to be implicated in tenosynovitis from overuse. Where only the tendons attached to the base of the thumb are affected, the condition is usually described as de Quervain's Syndrome.

Hand movement is controlled by two groups of muscles: The thenar muscle group and hypothenar group. These muscles are served by the motor branch of the median nerve with the exception of the powerful muscle surrounding the base of the thumb, which is supplied by the deep motor branch of the ulnar nerve. All of the hypothenar muscle group is supplied by the ulnar nerve, which enters the hand through the tunnel of Guyon, or Guyon's canal. A fine network of nerves provides further information to the long, ring, index, and little fingers, respectively.

HEAD, NECK, AND SHOULDERS

The muscles of the neck and shoulders are far larger and more powerful than those of the hand, and respond in a different way to repetitive work in the office. Their function is to support gross body movements, with the exception of the neck, which is capable of a wide range of subtle flexions. The neck muscles which suffer most from repetitive work are the sternomastoid, which runs down the side of the neck from the back of the base of the skull to the shoulder; the splenius, a deep-seated muscle running down the back of the neck; and the trapezius, a large muscle reaching all the way from the base of the skull to the middle of the spine. All these muscles are intricately bound up with the rhomboid and deltoid muscles of the shoulder, and pain in one is frequently indistinguishable from pain in another. Almost invariably, pain in these big muscles is the result of static tension rather than overuse.

Gross movement of the head is controlled by these same muscles; thus tension in muscles across the shoulder and down the back of the neck will almost certainly affect the head, usually in terms of headache. Other muscles of the head which are implicated in repetitive strain are the powerful masseter muscles of the jaw and the corrugator muscles across the forehead.

How RSI affects computer users

Repetitive strain injury is a *syndrome*—that is, a collection of symptoms most of which (but not necessarily all) will be present in the sufferer. It is characterized by numbness or tingling in the fingers; pain in the wrist, forearm, or shoulder when typing; discomfort when moving the mouse or depressing the mouse button, and aches and pains in the neck, shoulders, arms, elbows, and hands. It is also now one of the most widespread occupational disorders. In America, the Bureau of Labor Statistics recorded that RSI accounted for 65 percent of occupational illness in 1994, representing an alarming growth from just 21 percent in 1982.

Despite the prevalence of RSI since the start of the Industrial Revolution, it was not until 1980 that the term "repetitive strain injury" was called into being. It happened in Australia, following an apparent epidemic of musculoskeletal problems among office workers. The incidence of people reporting pain, tingling, and numbness of the upper limb began to increase dramatically in 1981 from its steady figure of between one and nine new patients per ten thousand, reaching a peak of six new patients per thousand office workers in 1987.

The sufferers presented many of the classical symptoms of tenosynovitis, an inflammation of the sheath surrounding the tendons of the wrist. This condition is relatively common among assembly line workers and is documented as a specific clinical condition but, in the Australian epidemic, things were not so straightforward. Other symptoms appeared regularly among sufferers—numbness, swelling, and complications affecting the neck and back—leading to panic reporting in the media of anything from stress-related health problems to mass hysteria even though the classic symptoms of tenosynovitis and carpal tunnel syndrome were not always present. At the time, the conditions reported were attributed to a psychological origin, with many commentators seeing the epidemic as the manifestation of social ills.

As the panic subsided, it became apparent that both psychological and physical factors were at work. Psychologically, many sufferers were experiencing work stress of the types described above or had little control over the nature of their jobs and the working environment. Others were simply hard-working. These conditions contributed to the gradual development of physical symptoms and the discovery of organic damage which led, in some cases, to severe and prolonged disability. The establishment of RSI as a distinct phenomenon, similar to but different from existing clinically documented conditions, has made it the subject of intense study ever since.

There are many afflictions which can be classified as repetitive strain injuries, although some of these do not appear in typists or computer keyboard users. Workers in heavy industry, for example, are more susceptible to injuries which affect the shoulder (humeral tendonitis). Tool users and tennis players are particularly prone (oddly enough) to tennis elbow or epicondylytis, a painful condition caused by repetitive extension of the wrists and fingers, which pulls on tendons attached to the elbow. Compression of the ulnar nerve, which runs from the elbow to the hand, is another musculoskeletal injury caused by repeated elbow flexion or leaning the elbows on hard surfaces for too long.

Clinical definitions of RSI usually refer to one of two specific forms: Carpal tunnel syndrome, and tenosynovitis (inflammation of the lubricating sheath around the tendon). Prior to the Australian epidemic, these two conditions were regarded as the sum total of RSIs, but it now appears that they comprise only a small minority (perhaps ten percent) of reported cases. A very large proportion of computer-related RSIs have no clinically defined symptoms at all but arise for reasons which simply cannot be pinned down with medical accuracy. For the sake of simplicity, some researchers classify carpal tunnel syndrome and tenosynovitis as "localized" RSI, while conditions with no apparent physical origin are referred to as "diffuse" RSI. This is primarily a semantic differentiation, but it has important implications for the theories of RSI which have emerged from different groups of researchers.

CARPAL TUNNEL SYNDROME

Carpal tunnel syndrome is one of the most common manifestations of RSI and also one of the best defined. Although present among non-computer users such as builders and professional tool users, it is now most prevalent among computer users.

The "carpal tunnel" is literally a tunnel, formed by the eight small carpal bones of the wrist and lined with a tough, fibrous layer. Through it pass the tendons of the finger flexor muscles, each wrapped in its own protective synovial sheath, and the median nerve. This nerve supplies sensation to the thumb, most of the palm, the index and middle fingers, and part of the ring finger. It also includes motor fibers which cause the muscles to contract in response to signals from the brain.

The first indication of carpal tunnel syndrome is numbness and tingling in the areas supplied by the median nerve—in many cases, the sensation is powerful enough to disturb the sufferer even during sleep. This gradually becomes more painful and develops into other uncomfortable sensations which may spread throughout the hand and up to the elbow. As the condition develops, pain and tingling continue throughout the day, and the patient may find it increasingly difficult to pick up and manipulate small objects. The muscles begin to waste and the affected limbs feel weak.

The symptoms of carpal tunnel syndrome are the result of impaired functioning of the median nerve (one of two nerves that serve the hand). When the median nerve is disturbed, the result can be reduced sensation in the thumb and first two fingers, or weakness of the muscle of the thumb, or both. These symptoms arise when the median nerve gets compressed where it passes through the carpal tunnel. In normal circumstances, ligaments, nerves, and tendons all function normally within the confines of the carpal tunnel. If the wrist is bent at an angle for many hours, many times a day; or if the tendons are engaged in fast, repetitive movements of the hand and fingers, pressure builds up in the tunnel. Overuse of the tendons causes their protective synovial sheath to swell, which in turn increases fluid pressure within the carpal tunnel and puts pressure directly on the median nerve. At first, the pressure affects the functioning of the nerve fibers by reducing the amount of blood reaching them. At this stage, the condition is curable with rest and avoidance of repetitive movements. Left untreated, the pressure in the wrist collapses the small blood vessels, reducing the blood supply to the supporting cells of the nerve fibers. Eventually, the insulating sheath on the nerve fibers is disrupted, and conduction of nerve impulses is slowed. In more severe cases, no conduction occurs at all. By this stage, the damage is irreparable and the patient will have reduced hand function for life.

Why do some people develop carpal tunnel syndrome while others in the same job don't? It is difficult to be precise, especially when the effects of unrelated stresses and strains play a part as well. One possible explanation is the anatomy of the wrist and relative dimensions of width and thickness. Individuals whose wrist thickness is less than 70 percent of wrist width ("wide" wrists) are far less likely to develop carpal tunnel syndrome than those in whom the balance is almost equal—that is, width and thickness are the same ("square" wrists).

Between 60 and 90 percent of sufferers are female. A number of things could explain this, primarily that much larger numbers of women are engaged in repetitive, detailed tasks (such as the precision placement of tiny components on circuit boards, typing, or sewing machine operation). It is probably significant that women tend to have smaller wrists than men, but more so that a number of predisposing physiological and medical conditions are more likely to be associated with carpal tunnel syndrome, and affect women only. Up to one in four women will report some symptoms of carpal tunnel syndrome during pregnancy, and estrogen-related factors such as oral contraceptives and premenstrual syndrome are also thought to be contributory factors. Diseases such as arthritis, gout, diabetes, tuberculosis, and hemophilia are more generally associated with the condition, and it can be provoked by traumas such as broken bones in the forearm, wrist, or hand.

The most common symptoms which doctors first see in a sufferer of carpal tunnel syndrome are numbness or tingling in the thumb and the two adjacent fingers, and pain, numbness, or other abnormal sensations in the hand at night. Although medical diagnosis depends heavily on the patient's report of symptoms, doctors also look for signs of shrinkage of the thick mound of muscle at the base of the thumb (the thenar eminence).

If it looks as if carpal tunnel syndrome may be responsible for the symptoms, a doctor may test nerve conduction, since this often provides a more reliable indication than the patient's report of symptoms. This method, both quick and relatively painless, involves electrophysiological tests to examine the conduction speed and amplitude of the nerve fibers via electrodes applied to the fingers, hand, and arm. Such a test will reveal whether impulses are traveling through the median nerve at the same rate as through the ulnar nerve (which also serves the hand, but does not pass through the carpal tunnel). In normal hands, the speed is the same. With carpal tunnel syndrome, the speed can be reduced by half, or more. Because this testing produces an objective measurement, it can be important in situations where, for example, an employer or insurance company does not believe the patient's report of symptoms.

Nerve conductance tests are not always entirely successful, so other techniques are being studied. The most promising avenues for research are vibrometry, or sensitivity to electrical stimulation, and visual techniques of inspecting the carpal tunnel. Vibrometry investigates the ability of the hand and fingers to sense vibration, a capability which is often impaired in carpal tunnel syndrome sufferers. It has a higher rate of problem detection than nerve conduction testing, but it also gives a positive result in a significant number of patients with no carpal tunnel problem. Authentic sufferers are also abnormally sensitive to low-level electrical stimulation in the affected hand, which could form the basis for a new test. For greater focus on the affected areas, some researchers are using magnetic resonance imaging literally to "see" the internal structure of the carpal tunnel and any abnormalities. If changes can be reliably found with this equipment, this approach could become an important diagnostic aid.

TENOSYNOVITIS

Also known as tenovaginitis, this disease describes the condition where the synovial sheath surrounding the tendons, particular those in the hand and lower arm, is inflamed. It is distinct from tendonitis (or peritendonitis) where only the surrounding tissue is inflamed, since no sheath is present. Tenosynovitis develops when overuse of the hand leads to swelling of the tendons and an increase in fluid pressure around the tendon sheath. Traces of the excess fluid seep into the tendon sheath, leading to fibrosis (excessive fibrous tissue) and adhesions, which may occur in conjunction with thickening or fraying of the tendon itself. As these conditions progress, the movement of the tendon within its sheath will become progressively more difficult and painful, at which point the condition becomes known as stenosing tenosynovitis.

The primary cause of tenosynovitis is thought to be muscular overuse and accompanying circulatory changes. Symptoms begin with a dull ache across the areas involved—typically the tendons of the thumb and forefinger—which becomes worse when the hand is used to perform small, repetitive movements. Eventually grip weakens and the pain may become sharper, with swelling developing around the thumb and fingers. In advanced cases, an audible sound accompanies movement, described as a crunching noise.

Tenosynovitis is one of the few upper limb disorders to have the dubious distinction of official classification as an industrial disease (in the United Kingdom). Typists have always been disproportionately affected by it and this has increased since the introduction of electronic keyboards, possibly because the elimination of the carriage return handle has also eliminated the only rest typists ever get.

NON-PATHOLOGICAL RSI

By far the most common and the most mysterious condition, non-pathological RSI (also referred to as diffuse RSI) has no clear physical manifestation but makes up some 80-90 percent of all cases. Sufferers report symptoms similar to those of carpal tunnel syndrome, including sharp pains in the wrist, stiffness and pain in the fingers, and unpleasant tingling sensations running the full length of the arm. The whole area may be sensitive to touch. If the patient has had the symptoms for some time, they may persist indefinitely, even if he or she has abandoned all efforts to use a keyboard. The lack of physical signs indicating a real disease has made it difficult for sufferers of this version of RSI to gain sympathy and support, as evidenced by the controversial court cases described earlier. Yet it remains one of the most serious and most prevalent health threats to which modern workers are currently exposed.

HEADACHE, NECK-ACHE, AND SHOULDER PAIN

Although not strictly the result of repetitive motion, the most frequently remarked musculoskeletal disorders arising directly from the constant use of the computer are headaches, neck-aches, and shoulder pain. General musculoskeletal aches and pains are a common feature of computer use, with many formal and informal studies quoting a daily occurrence of headache, neck, and shoulder pain in 10 to 50 percent of computer users on any given day. The proportion of people reporting such discomfort rises as hours spent in front of a computer increase, and symptoms become more severe as exposure becomes more prolonged. In order to classify these as distinct, work-related complaints, it is becoming more common to classify broader musculoskeletal ailments in the same bracket as the specific hand and wrist RSIs.

Of all the disorders that plague computer users, the humble headache has to be among the most common and persistent. Where no pathological condition is present (such as tumor, inflammation, or infection), headache is most commonly due to muscular tension around the head and neck, which may become severe if it is allowed to accumulate. Like many health-related disturbances, stress is often the originating factor in headaches. For the average computer user, stress originates as a general consequence of computer work and can lead to headache if other factors are present. Typically, these will be screen glare, poorly placed lighting, and, most importantly, prolonged concentration on a computer screen. Some people tend to squint or frown when concentrating, while others clench or grind their teeth—each of these behaviors causes a different type of headache. Those who frown often develop pain above the eyes, where the muscles have been most fiercely clenched. Teeth-grinders tense the large muscles of the jaw, creating pain and tension around the ear and temple, and squinters suffer from headaches which are generally indistinguishable from eyestrain. The muscle groups involved in headaches usually "refer" pain to other areas, such as the temple, behind the eyes, and the neck. Sometimes, sufferers will develop sore, reddened eyes and interpret their symptoms as more serious than they are.

Along with headache, tension and stiffness in the neck and shoulders are all too common to computer users. Neck and shoulder pain arise from the unnaturally still position many users assume when in front of the screen, often for hours at a time. Repetitive, monotonous work is particularly to blame, and tension in the neck is more likely where the screen reflects too much light or glare. Hunched shoulders, curved spine, and craned neck are characteristic of repetitive computer work, as are the musculoskeletal problems which follow.

How computers lead to RSI

In concise terms, Ramazzini's early observations identified the principal cause of repetitive strain injury—fixed posture, repetitive motion, and psychological stress. All of these are overwhelmingly present for the computer user, and in many ways it seems a miracle that so few people develop RSI. What is it about these three components that implicates them?

FIXED POSTURE

The human body is designed to move. Nerves deep within the muscles provide constant information about the stretch and movement within each muscle, and a complex network of tendons and ligaments controls our gross body movements as well as fine control. Movement maintains the flow of blood and lymph around the circulatory system and provides the muscles with exercise, which in turn maintains muscle and general health.

Many twentieth-century occupations are sedentary, and this in itself has given rise to a general increase in health concerns regarding exercise, weight, and overall fitness. Computer usage is also a sedentary activity, but it demands a level of concentration which few other desk-based jobs can match. Partly because of the activity on the screen, and partly because of the reduced need for gross body movements (turning, reaching, or standing), movement is reduced to eye tracking, small movements of the hand and wrist, and small inclinations of the head. The nature and detail of information displayed on the screen can be absorbing; computer users can become transfixed at their desks and may remain almost motionless for hours at a time.

A static, seated posture is not natural for the human body, and forces many muscles out of their normal resting state into one of static posture maintenance. Although nerve fibers alert the mind when muscles are held tense in an unnatural attitude for too long, it is possible that high levels of stimulation from the computer might override or ignore these signals. This lack of low-level, natural movement and adjustment eventually leads to the aches and stiffness that characterize the headache, neck, and shoulder pain described above.

During computer use, the body assumes a constrained and unnatural posture. The position of the head becomes fixed so that uninterrupted viewing of the screen is possible. The hands, arms, fingers, and trunk are arranged around the machine and furniture; and muscle tension throughout the neck, shoulders, and upper body increases through visual strain, mental load, and adaptation to posture. Initially, prolonged muscular tension and static posture produce acute fatigue and pain in the muscles concerned—usually the neck and shoulder muscles feel it first. During initial usage, the pain and tension will generally clear up within a few hours of leaving the computer. If the posture is regularly maintained over a long period, however, the pain may become more permanent.

Some researchers have used a technique called electromyography to record the muscular activity of the shoulders during prolonged bouts of typing. In all cases, the activity was least when people were relaxed; levels increased to a peak of activity during intensive typing. The electrical activity revealed by the electromyograph indicates the greatest proportional increase in tension in the muscles responsible for lifting the shoulders and upper arms. The tension in itself is uncomfortable and can cause prolonged damage; but its indirect effect is the distortion of alignment of the arm, wrist, and hand—and increased likelihood of an injury such as carpal tunnel syndrome.

Neck pain (and often, consequently, headache) also begins gradually as a result of fixed staring at a small area or glancing repeatedly from one to another (from the screen to a source document, for example). Pain and muscular fatigue become apparent more rapidly when the head is held at an extreme angle to the neck for a prolonged period, anything greater than 15 degrees. This happens if the object of attention lies outside the normal line of sight, causing excessive craning or inclination of the neck. "Normal" line of sight means 10 degrees beneath the horizontal. Gaze straight ahead, head and neck in a natural posture, then drop your line of vision just slightly—this is the normal line of vision. Anything which lies outside this range will cause you to hold your head and neck in an unnatural posture. Gazing directly ahead or slightly upwards tilts the head too far back, compressing and tensing the muscles at the base of the skull. Gazing to the left or right twists the neck out of alignment and exerts an uneven strain on the neck muscles; and gazing downwards shifts the center of gravity forward to the head, exerting a greater strain on the lower neck and shoulder muscles which tense up to compensate. Fixed posture is therefore primarily responsible for musculoskeletal complaints of the head, neck, and shoulders, rather than the more specific afflictions of the hand and wrist.

REPETITIVE MOTION

What is it about repetition that is so harmful to our health? In the above examples of muscular pain in the neck and shoulders, the pain is a consequence of static tension. The muscles are held in a single, motionless position for far longer than is normal, causing stiffness and ache. Repetitive movement, surely, should allow the muscles the movement they need? This is not, of course, the case. Of all the muscle types in the human body, cardiac muscle (the heart) is the only type which is designed to be in use all the time. It possesses many unique properties, including high levels of elasticity, its own blood supply, and an untiring ability to contract and pump more than once a second for the entire life span of a human being. No other muscle is equipped to perform like this.

Non-cardiac muscles all operate in the same basic way—that is, they are either resting or working. Muscles begin to work when they receive nerve impulses from the brain, at which point a complex biochemical process takes place. The "excited" muscle tenses up (shortens) and converts available chemical energy (derived from food) into mechanical energy (movement) and heat. This energy store is composed of a chemical called glycogen, a simple carbohydrate which resides in the muscles at all times. During intensive or prolonged activity (such as physical exercise), the process of converting glycogen to energy relies on the aerobic metabolic process, in which oxygen is used to break down the glycogen into carbon dioxide and water. If the pace is sustained, other chemicals such as fat and protein are included in the process.

At low intensities, the muscles are able to operate using just the immediate store of energy available to them. If the demand for muscle activity is not great (as in typing, for example), the muscles derive energy by simply splitting the glucose molecules into two atoms of lactic acid, without requiring oxygen. This is known as anaerobic processing. Anaerobic processing sounds like less

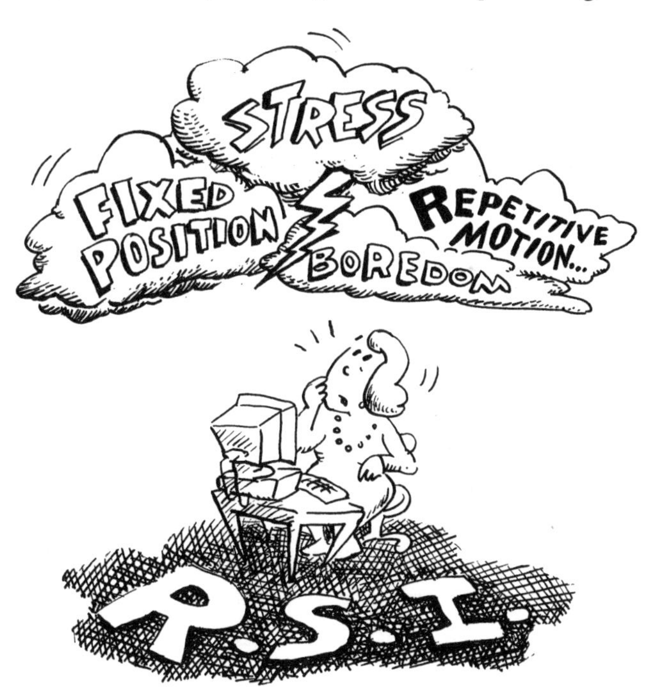

How computer use can lead to RSI.

effort, but is actually more tiring in some ways. This is because lactic acid is a by-product of anaerobic processing, which builds up in the muscles until high levels of acidity begin to interfere with muscular contractions—the sensation known as fatigue.

Muscular fatigue is a precursor of repetitive strain injury. It is not a direct cause, but muscles which are tired from constant use in a repetitive sequence are more likely to be used in an unhealthy way. For example, prolonged keyboard use will create sensations of general fatigue in the hand, wrist, and forearm, encouraging the untrained typist to rest his or her arms flat on the table. This may relieve the fatigue, but it forces the typist to flex the wrists at a relatively acute angle to reach the keys. It is this flexing which leads directly to pinching and compression of the tendons and ultimately, tenosynovitis and carpal tunnel syndrome.

PSYCHOLOGICAL STRESS AND BOREDOM

It has already been shown that stress is an increasing phenomenon in our daily lives and even more so in the office: How does it affect our susceptibility to RSI?

The link is unclear and there is probably not a simple or direct relationship, but stress undoubtedly contributes to the development of RSI in some individuals. Many keyboard users lack formal training in typing skills and thus begin intensive typing work from a position of anxiety, perhaps fearing that they lack the skills and ability to perform the job for which they are being paid. Without the training required, they tend to rely on just two or three fingers to type, imposing an additional strain on those fingers and the tendons which must be stretched farther than normal to reach all the keys. Other keyboard users may have gained their skills on the relatively non-technical typewriter, and perceive the computer as frightening complex technology which threatens their livelihood. In either case, such users approach computer use with high levels of anxiety, and often have little control over the tasks they must perform. Still other employees may have conquered their fear of the computer but still experience high levels of work-related stress. To understand this, it is important to be aware that the physiological stress reaction does not have to be in response to high-energy panic and work overload. In fact, you are just as likely to feel stressed when you are bored or understimulated.

Boredom can be regarded as the physiological response to monotony. *Monotony* describes the basic circumstances in which we get bored, but does not explain what boredom is. From a human point of view, monotony is a state of understimulation, and boredom is a complex mental state characterized by decreased activity in the higher nervous centers, weariness, lethargy, and diminished alertness. People get most bored most quickly when they do prolonged, repetitive work which is not very difficult but demands some sort of concentration. Typing a lengthy or technical prewritten document is a good example. The actions of typing such a document are prolonged and repetitive, but because the typist is simply required to copy existing text, no real thought is required. On the other hand, the typist needs to keep an eye on things to ensure that subheadings are bold, commas correctly inserted, and that no spelling mistakes slip through. In other words, the typist doesn't need to think about the job in an intellectual way, but nor can he or she think about anything else.

Boredom also sets in during prolonged, repetitive work which calls for continuous vigilance. For example, the job may be to inspect all the chips on printed circuit boards in a factory, just before they are packed, to check that none are damaged. The chances of one being damaged, after many previous checks, are so remote that it almost never happens. But if it happens, just once, and a faulty board gets through, your entire company could fail vital quality control tests, and it would be your fault. So even though you are looking for something that will probably never happen, you cannot relax and think about anything else, even for a moment.

When someone is bored, a number of physiological events take place: With no input via the senses, nervous impulses to the brain simply dry up. The higher, thinking parts of the brain become progressively less active, and eventually learn to accept the monotonous situation as normal. When this occurs, the broader nervous system slows down too, reducing your ability to think and react. That's why it is so difficult to begin work when it arrives, even when you have had nothing to do all day. Like unused muscles, the thinking centers of the brain atrophy if they are not used regularly. Boredom is often associated with feelings of sleepiness, weariness, or lethargy—usually this is most likely to occur after a heavy meal, or in a warm, stuffy environment. Those workers without such luxuries may experience boredom as intense dissatisfaction, frustration, or irritation. Time seems to drag and minutes seem like hours. Everything feels like a chore.

The repetitive activities and static posture described above are part of and ultimately lead to boredom and psychological stress. Intense boredom, a lack of control over job task, and almost no opportunity to think creatively all generate tension and misery, which increase vulnerability to RSI. Muscular tension derived from frustration increases the resistance against which the tendons and nerves of the carpal tunnel have to press; not to mention the intense shoulder, neck, and head pains of repetitive work. More subtly, the pain of repetitive injuries may be felt sooner by a bored individual than a fulfilled one—the bored one has little else to think about, after all.

Different opinions about RSI

Most theorists agree that the elements described above are all present to some extent in sufferers of RSI. Exactly what the individual contribution of each element is, and how it interacts with the others, remain the subject of ferocious debate.

THE HYSTERICAL VIEW

At one extreme is the view that RSI simply does not exist. No one is arguing that work is never stressful, and clearly there are well-defined medical conditions which we can call RSI. What about a more scientific point of view? Isn't it possible, as some employers believe, that RSI is just a concoction for lazy people who need a reliable excuse to get them out of work? To many people, this controversial point of view is the only "real" explanation of RSI. Since RSI has no organic origin in bacteria, virus, or other microbe, and since it cannot be seen and not all computer or keyboard users get it, how can we describe it as a real illness?

Groups who hold this view tend to require proof in order to perform *their* work. Employers and insurance companies need hard evidence in order to provide the financing and benefits normally required of illness; other adherents include a minority of orthopedic surgeons—medically qualified doctors specializing in the treatment of bone and muscle injuries. The argument of these groups is simple: With the exceptions of carpal tunnel syndrome, tenosynovitis, and other variations of localized injury to the upper limb, there is absolutely no physical evidence for RSI. It cannot, therefore, exist.

It is not uncommon for sufferers of RSI to exhibit no clinical symptoms whatsoever—in fact it is surprisingly common. In the first real "epidemic" in the early 1980s, *less than five percent* of reported cases of RSI were officially diagnosed as carpal tunnel syndrome, epicondylytis (tennis elbow), or tenosynovitis. The remaining 95 percent showed no objective symptoms from radiological, vascular, electrodiagnostic, pathological, or other physiological test. This extraordinary imbalance between measurable illness and absence from work rapidly led to the labeling of RSI as "the shirker's disease," and its victims as lazy. What made it different, however, was the extent and duration of the cases. Unlike other documented cases of hysterical or conversion illness, RSI remained a distressing condition in many people for many months. Since the implication of the hysterical view is that all sufferers of diffuse RSI (for whatever reasons) fabricate their complaints, its supporters have modified their views to acknowledge the influence of psychological factors. Proponents now accept that RSI sufferers do experience pain and weakness, but propose that this is the result of psychogenic factors—in other words, RSI is all in the mind. They attribute the symptoms to a combination of anxiety, lack of confidence in one's ability to do the job, paranoia, and general frustration with the working environment, all of which are expressed as RSI. As far as the hysterical view is concerned, RSI is, at best, the painful manifestation of mental anxiety and, at worst, an attempt to beat the system.

THE PHYSIOLOGICAL VIEW

In direct opposition to the hysterical view is the physiological view, widely held by physical therapists, whose research efforts have been largely directed towards evidence for a physiological basis underlying *all* cases of RSI. They acknowledge the physiological distinctions between the clinical status of carpal tunnel syndrome and diffuse RSI, but argue that the difference is just a matter of degree. The root cause, physiological research suggests, is a phenomenon called *adverse mechanical tension.* During prolonged, repetitive movement, the muscles become tense and nerve fibers more active. According to the theory of adverse mechanical tension, if muscle tension persists the nerves may become entrapped between muscle fibers, giving rise to painful sensations which go on for hours after work has stopped. In severe cases, it can affect many sites across the body, including the shoulders, neck, and back as well as the upper limbs. The pain creates a vicious circle of tension and further nerve entrapment and the effect is the sensation of RSI. Adverse mechanical tension gains support from physical therapists who have used stretching and manipulating techniques to free nerves, with good results.

More traditional physiologically-oriented researchers believe there is a close physical link between psychological discomfort and ill-health of all kinds. These groups suggest that a stressful environment leads to the subjective experience of unhappiness or helplessness. This experience triggers hormonal and biochemical changes in the brain which lead to the secretion of excessive quantities of certain chemicals, which in turn lead to feelings of depression (itself a complex and poorly understood condition). Depression is associated with a decline in the activity of the immune system, which increases a person's vulnerability to all sorts of illnesses. Alternatively, anxiety may be the predominant emotion, in which case the sufferer may become tense and irritable. These feelings are associated with a parallel increase in blood pressure, increased secretion of stomach acid and a greater vulnerability to heart attacks or stomach ulcers. The result is a stressed, unhappy individual who is more likely to experience and report subjective feelings of pain, headache, and associated symptoms of RSI.

THE PSYCHOLOGICAL/PSYCHOANALYTIC VIEW

Psychologists believe that the roots of RSI lie within our minds, although this does not imply that the final manifestation of the disease is any less real than a broken bone. Repetitive strain injury first came to the attention of psychological thinkers when it was no more than a humble writer's cramp.

Documented since Ramazzini's time in the early eighteenth century, writer's cramp affected clerks and "scriveners" (scribes), giving rise to its old name "scrivener's palsy." It seems natural to expect that prolonged writing with a quill would cause muscular fatigue and pain in the writing hand, and indeed this was a common complaint among the educated classes of the eighteenth and nineteenth centuries. With the advent of Freudian thinking in the early twentieth century, however, writer's cramp came under the scrutiny of far more sophisticated theorists. The tense gripping action of the hand during writing was attributed to repressed anger, and the deterioration of writing action to "neurological breakdown." In the first flush of the discovery of the unconscious, psychoanalysts paid scant attention to dull explanations such as the awkward shape of the pen, or the sheer effort of writing with one for prolonged periods.

Our understanding of non-organic illness began with the work of Sigmund Freud, the famous psychologist and psychoanalyst. Based on his work with patients in late nineteenth-century Vienna, he put together the first comprehensive theory of the unconscious. Briefly, Freud argued that experiences which were unpleasant when they occurred are forgotten—or repressed. We may think we have forgotten them, but in fact they remain in the unconscious mind. Abnormal or irrational fear of certain situations or things can often be traced to these repressed memories. For example, someone's irrational fear of dogs may ultimately be traced back to an incident when a dog attacked or bit the person. They may have no recollection of the attack since it was unpleasant and the memory repressed, but it clearly affects them in their everyday life. Freud treated people with such fears by uncovering the repressed memory and bringing it from the unconscious into the conscious mind. Once such memories are recognized and acknowledged, Freud believed, they cease to exert an influence over our lives and behavior.

The basic premise of the unconscious and its influence on our behavior underlies much of modern psychoanalysis. Different practitioners take different perspectives and use different treatments, but all share a common understanding that experiences which we cannot recall or recognize affect our lives, often on a deep level.

Illness as avoidance

The mechanism by which unhappy memories and experiences are translated into physical ailments, behaviors, or "neuroses" is complex and poorly understood. At one extreme, Freud and his followers might argue that physical or behavioral disorders bear a direct relationship to the real experience which underlies them. For example, Freud believed that individuals who had witnessed or overheard a scene about which they felt guilty or distressed were more likely to develop "hysterical blindness" (or deafness, sore throat, headache, paralysis, and a wide range of minor conditions). Such people generally lost their sight although no organic damage to their eyes could be found. Freud originally interpreted such illnesses as a form of self-inflicted punishment or shield, arguing that the unconscious mind had used its unpleasant repressed memories to construct a suitable way of avoiding the distressing memory.

Modern psychoanalysts refer to such conditions as "conversion illness," which describes the conversion of a mental anxiety into a physical illness, such that the physical illness conceals the mental anxiety and also enables the "sufferer" to benefit. For example, Freud might argue that anxiety about public speaking might manifest itself as a sore throat or loss of speech. Or, if there is a possibility that a skin rash may provide a better way of avoiding a speaking engagement (if cameras are involved, for example), then it is more likely that such anxiety will be manifested as a rash. In the case of RSI, the symptoms are seen primarily as a manifestation of generalized occupational anxiety; and secondarily as a means of achieving financial compensation.

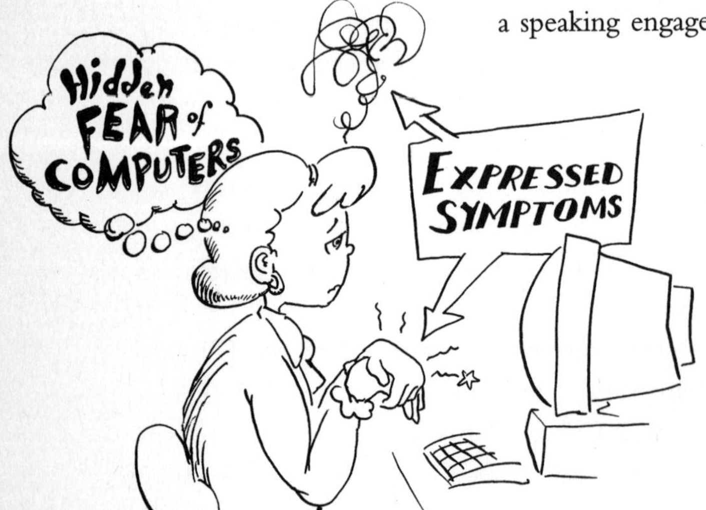

Freud's conception of the conscious and unconscious mind, and how they interact.

Illness as an expression of anxiety

Illnesses which arise from mental or emotional disturbances are called psychosomatic illnesses, where *psycho* means "of the mind" and *soma* means "of the body." In effect, mental anxiety is expressed as a physical illness. Psychosomatic illness differs from conversion illness in that a psychosomatic condition is more likely to be related to an existing physical weakness than to a situational difficulty—thus pain in the wrist may not be a reflection of a dread of typing so much as real pain in an already damaged part of the body. The links are so complex and wide-ranging that some doctors and psychiatrists believe that all illness is somehow related to the state of the mind. Some eastern medical philosophies are based on the notion that illness is *always* and *only* the result of emotional disturbance, and that the correction of such disturbance is the only cure. The research into the links between our state of mind and body is vast, and to go into it in depth would certainly take more space than is available here. What does seem to be beyond dispute, however, is that mental health does have some bearing on physical health. In simple terms, people who are generally happy and fulfilled tend to be healthier than those who are unhappy, frustrated, or bored. Some illnesses may be the manifestation of a deeper discontent, while others may be the result of increased vulnerability to viruses, bacteria, and fatigue. Either way, it is impossible to disregard the influence of our emotional and mental health when considering the cause of, or cure for, work-related illness.

The socio-occupational view

Broader theories view the individual's immediate working environment as a crucial factor in susceptibility to RSI. This applies equally to physiological factors and psychological factors, seeing these as meaningful only in the context of the environment. For example, one of the few "facts" of RSI is that women suffer from it more than men. Research suggests that women develop RSI anywhere from two to ten times more frequently than men, and indeed, gender seems to be the only reliable predictor of who gets RSI. In carpal tunnel syndrome—and in other musculoskeletal complaints of the hand and wrist as well—peculiarly feminine issues seem to correlate with RSI. Women's smaller wrists are more vulnerable than men's, but this appears to be exacerbated by factors such as pregnancy, the use of oral contraceptives, menopause, and gynecological surgery. The exact mechanism by which one affects the other is unclear, if indeed it exists at all. Hormonal changes brought on by these conditions are known to alter the flexibility of the ligaments, tendency of blood to clot, or levels of water retention in the soft tissues. Whether this has any bearing at all on susceptibility to RSI is quite simply not known. If may be that these factors correlate with incidents of RSI only because they also correlate with some other, unknown factor. There are certainly plenty of contenders.

A prime suspect which correlates with being female and having RSI is the cluster of working characteristics commonly labeled "job dissatisfaction." While it might be argued that job dissatisfaction is a result rather than a cause of RSI, it also seems likely that dissatisfaction encourages workers to report RSI earlier in its development, and more frequently. The computer has changed the work practices of many organizations, invariably to "increase productivity." These practices now include fewer staff, heavier workloads, more specialized (less diverse) tasks, and a greater output of work. Not only are these practices inherently harmful in that they increase levels of repetitive work, but they also reduce an employee's personal involvement in the job. Lack of control and involvement has already been shown to contribute directly to stress, and stress is clearly related to dissatisfaction.

Increasingly, we have intensive, technology-driven work practices which demand greater effort while squeezing out individual thought and initiative—the result is repetition and boredom. Many companies demand a minimum keying rate which forces employees to type far faster and for longer periods than they otherwise would. Other companies do not demand but encourage this practice by offering pay bonuses for employees who meet minimum data entry targets. Such practices obviously entail prolonged, rapid, or forceful repetitive motions leading to fatigue of all the muscles involved. Without such demands or incentives, high-frequency keyboard users such as programmers are better able to judge when to stop or pause. They are also far more in control of their workload, have greater involvement, and often take a personal interest in its progress.

So which came first, the low-status, unstimulating tasks or the physically demanding, repetitive typing which accompanies them? The answer is not important—what matters is that the two occur together in nearly all cases of diffuse RSI. Is RSI, therefore, the combined effect of physical overload and psychological underload? Even here the answer is not clear cut. Highly motivated employees engaged in stimulating work which they enjoy still develop RSI, while others employed in boring, menial tasks do not. This implies that the physiological factors described earlier (wrist dimensions, water retention, or other medical interactions) probably have some influence. On average, however, employees working on menial, pressured tasks are more likely to develop RSI than employees who control and enjoy their work. It seems likely that there is some psychosomatic effect behind the development of RSI, even if it is not an absolute prerequisite.

Other work-related factors

We have seen that stress and boredom can exacerbate muscular tension, which in turn can increase the susceptibility of some individuals to carpal tunnel syndrome and other clinically defined illnesses of the hand and wrist. The interesting cases are those incidences of RSI where no such clinical condition is present. The physiology and psychology of stress and boredom are clearly implicated in the development of RSI, and their influence may, in fact, be the most likely reason why some people get RSI while others, performing similar tasks, do not. It is certainly difficult to explain some cases of RSI without reference to non-organic factors. Typically, inexplicable diseases, rashes, and complaints which arise psychosomatically disappear within a matter of days (even hours). Repetitive strain injury, however, appears to endure well beyond the moment when it can be explained away as a "hysterical" reaction. What else, then, can explain the lack of symptoms.

In an extended Australian research project, cases of diffuse RSI were investigated in the context of the wider environment. The most striking observation was the high incidence of RSI in computer keyboard users compared to that of traditional typewriter users. This observation seems particularly strange given the relatively intensive effort some typewriters require, especially when compared to electronic keyboards. The research suggested that it was the incessant typing on an electronic keyboard, rather than hard key presses, that laid the foundations for RSI. Typewriters, particularly manual ones, force their users into taking regular breaks from the action of typing. Hitting the carriage return, changing paper, or adjusting margins seem to be trivial tasks, but even such minor efforts break the routine of typing. These breaks appear to have a significant effect on the prevention of RSI, far more so than the effort required to depress the keys. Different movements rest and exercise different areas of the hand, reducing the strain on a single set of muscles and tendons. Conventional typewriters require more wrist movement and less finger extension than electronic ones, limiting pressure on the median and ulnar nerves and placing less strain on the finger ligaments.

Taken to an extreme, it is not just electronic keyboards which force workers into a repetitive and monotonous task. The whole concept of office automation has created a culture of increased productivity, encouraging managers to seek more and more output from their employees. Available computing power now exceeds the capabilities of its human operators, putting the pressure on people to keep up. When computers instead of filing cabinets are used to store files, it is no longer necessary to have someone walk to a filing cabinet to retrieve a document. Instead, they can find it in the computer by navigating through the file structure with a keyboard. If that same keyboard reduces the number of breaks a person must take to maintain files, for instance, it is a simple step to the next stage for employers—replace those breaks with more typing. In the Australian study, it was thought reasonable for employees to demand 14,000 keystrokes per hour if the power was available. Many of the companies surveyed also programmed their computers to monitor the inputting rate of employees and report on those whose work dropped below the given rate. (It is not difficult to imagine the tense work atmosphere that was created!)

The widespread use of minimum keystroke requirements would imply a higher than five percent rate of "real" (that is, clinically defined) RSI. It also implies that countries across the world should be experiencing RSI epidemics on the scale of the Australian one. In neither case is this true. Programmers and novelists (both prolific keyboard users) do not routinely suffer from RSI; and although RSI is generally on the rise, no other country has reported an "epidemic" in the way Australia has. There must be other, wider reaching social factors which lie behind the Australian epidemic.

THE COMBINED THEORY OF RSI

The growing complexity and sophistication of our knowledge of RSI makes all of these views interesting—but somewhat unsatisfactory. Clearly, they each have something to offer, but is it helpful to regard one view as "correct" and the others as "wrong"? Obviously not: Even the most radical of the current theories of RSI are based on specific notions of causality, but like so many theories of complex phenomena, they cannot account for everything. What is required is a coherent theory which acknowledges the physiological and psychological elements of the disease, describes the mechanism of their interaction and discusses their integration within a social and occupational framework.

The first attempt at a comprehensive theory of RSI has been put forth in an Australian study conducted in 1992 by Cohen and colleagues. In their paper, the researchers argued for the combined influence of physical overuse, postural problems, psychogenic anxieties, and stress-related psychosomatic manifestations in the development of RSI. Most significantly, the study suggests that prolonged muscle overuse in an environment like the one described above can lead to permanent changes in the functioning of the central nervous system. In a healthy individual, the skin and muscles of the arm have a rich supply of touch receptors, dotted with pain receptors. Sufferers of RSI, it appears, have a disproportionately high concentration of pain receptors, suggesting that the function of some touch receptors actually changes to that of a pain receptor. This could explain the gradual development of pain from a temporary nuisance into a permanent condition.

Cohen's work suggests that the only safe conclusion to be drawn about RSI is that it is the result of many factors (some of which may still be unknown) interacting in a complex and poorly understood way. Our current understanding traces RSI most directly to the quality of work life. A vague term, this nevertheless describes the spectrum of causes: General work stress, lack of control over job content, pressure (implicit or explicit) to meet unreasonable data input targets, repetitive motion, monotony, poor career prospects, and awareness of work-related health issues. This mix of factors translates both directly and indirectly into a range of health problems: Musculoskeletal aches and pains, boredom, tension, muscle fatigue, depression, suppression of the immune system and increased susceptibility to minor illness, unhappiness and negative feelings about work in general. RSI has direct links to some of these practices (repetitive motion and data input targets, for example); and indirect links to others (boredom and depression). It is not always possible to track the incidence of RSI either, as the inexplicable and isolated epidemic in Australia shows. Even reporting RSI to your employer depends on a range of factors, such as the extent to which RSI is socially acceptable; the likelihood of getting another, equally paid job without keyboard skills; and the fear of being labeled lazy or incurable and therefore of no further use.

Summary

Clearly the number of people who fake RSI is negligible: They have a lot to lose and almost nothing to gain, so what's the point? The conclusion must be, first, that a relatively small number of people develop well-documented, clinically defined ailments of the hand, wrist, and arm as a direct result of prolonged computer keyboard use. A far larger number, however, develop the same symptoms of pain, weakness, and debility without exhibiting any observable or measurable physical damage. It may be that there are very different reasons behind the development of carpal tunnel syndrome and diffuse RSI; or it may be that one is simply a more severe manifestation of the other.

Cynics have taken the view that diffuse RSI is used as an excuse to leave by employees who are bored with their jobs. Since so many cases of RSI have no observable signs, they argue, it is easy for disenchanted workers to claim they have the disease, receive medical certification, and remain off work indefinitely on sick pay. If one employee succeeds, others will soon follow until the entire "epidemic" becomes traceable to a single incident. This "mass hysteria" relies on several elements being present. Where general stresses and strains are part of a tedious typing job, the argument runs, workers are more likely to experience low-level aches and pains as a result of tension and postural problems. If this is combined with a conviction that such work is damaging to the hands and wrists, and the observation that other employees have received medical certification without "proving" an illness, it is far more likely that other employees will develop—or appear to develop—RSI.

This is a powerful but flawed argument. Powerful, because social acceptability and the behavior of others (particularly friends and relatives) *is* a strong influence on other types of behavior. But flawed, because it is impossible to disentangle cause and effect in social behavior, but it is almost certainly true that they feed off one another in a cycle.

The isolated RSI epidemic in Australia has often been explained in this way and, purely because it was so isolated, may be partly true. It is not uncommon for healthy people to develop feelings of faints and nausea when visiting a hospital, or to feel sick at the sight of an airplane paper bag. Through a process of empathy (awareness of another's feelings) and association (of hospitals or sick bags with illness and nausea), it is quite natural to experience the symptoms one observed in others, albeit temporarily. (As a case in point, the author developed the unmistakable symptoms of RSI during the writing of this chapter, which faded when studying the chapter on "Prevention and Cure.") As people observe others performing some behavioral ritual (be it cohabitation, air sickness, or RSI) they are more likely to perform it themselves, eventually turning it into a routine and acceptable element of social behavior. (This thinking underlies many of the arguments linking TV violence with increasing real life violence, where increased exposure to a particular attitude or behavior ultimately makes it more acceptable.) Some sufferers of RSI during the Australian epidemic may have experienced symptoms for these reasons, which led to the increased acceptability of RSI as a legitimate illness. This still does not explain why the symptoms persisted for so long after sufferers left the environment where the complaint developed.

The argument that RSI sufferers are lazy implies that symptoms are deliberately faked by sufferers for gain. A decline in the rate of RSI, such people believe, is related only to the increased difficulty of getting a different job (during a recession, for example). So what exactly do they stand to gain? At face value, indefinite sick pay and no work seems ideal, but this is rarely the outcome. Few companies are altruistic enough to provide health compensation schemes which allow sick employees to be paid indefinitely; at some point, payment will cease and the employee be legitimately dismissed. During a recession, although actual cases do decline, informal evidence suggests that this is simply because more people are tolerating the pain. Fear of losing their job and failing to find another keeps many sufferers silent, and the effects of such a reaction will only become apparent in the long term. Sufferers of RSI lose social contacts, independence, and the chance to gain experience. Ploughing through the legal system to secure compensation is traumatic in its own way, and the amounts secured are rarely worth the tremendous effort. Faking RSI is simply not worth it.

The more we study RSI and its causes, the more apparent it becomes that our understanding is patchy. Statistics may lead us towards one conclusion, but there are always exceptions which prevent these conclusions from becoming accepted as facts. RSI, even when it has well-defined symptoms, has become a quantifiable (and therefore socially acceptable) outlet for a whole range of non-specific work concerns. This does not mean it is fraudulent, but simply that current working practices, particularly computer-related, can be harmful to our health in the broadest sense. Stepping back from the specific links between work and RSI, it seems fair to describe it as a classic example of a twentieth-century disease, combining direct physiological, complex psychological, and broad occupational factors in a single condition. RSI cannot, therefore, be understood, treated, or prevented in isolation. It can only be dealt with in the context of social, technological, and economic factors which are themselves currently undergoing a period of dramatic change.

CHAPTER 4

Electromagnetism and the Computing Environment

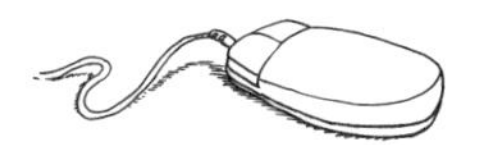

INTERACTING WITH COMPUTERS may well be a hazardous business, but if you pay attention to your posture and take regular breaks from the keyboard, it must be fairly safe, surely? The answer is "yes," "no," and "we don't know." Yes, there is no real evidence that it is anything but safe if you use a computer in a sensible, balanced way. No, although there's nothing the naked eye can see, computers generate electromagnetic fields which are known to affect the normal function of living cells. We don't know—whether these emissions have any effect on human tissues, or what the consequences of exposure are, if there are any at all.

What is electromagnetism?

Electromagnetic radiation is a form of one of the fundamental forces of the universe: *Electromagnetism*. In its natural state, electromagnetism comprises both magnetic fields and electrical charge which combine to form electromagnetic waves. The two types of fields—electrical and magnetic—are related and arise from the same phenomena, but they have individual distinguishing characteristics. Electric fields generate a potential (a voltage), are measured in millivolts or volts per meter, and are relatively easy to shield against by using conductive materials. Magnetic fields generate a current (amperage). These fields are measured in milliamps per meter or sometimes in related units of gauss, and are difficult to shield against. Electromagnetic waves are generated every time electricity or magnetism changes direction or strength. Since electricity is just the movement of electrons, and electrons are part of every atom that surrounds us, we are constantly bathed in a low level of EM radiation. Natural varieties include light, infrared, and ultraviolet, cosmic rays from distant exploding stars, and radio signals from thunderstorms. Most modern technology relies on or produces electromagnetic radiation—radio, TV, microwave, and X-ray are all examples.

Electromagnetic radiation constantly varies in strength from zero to the maximum level of a particular signal and back again. The speed at which it does this defines the frequency, and thus the effects, of the radiation. A *frequency of zero* means the field is not moving at all—this is called an *electrostatic* field, in other words, a field where the electrons are static. Just above zero are the slowest forms of genuine electromagnetic radiation, called *extremely low frequency* (ELF) and *very low frequency* (VLF) radiation respectively. These have a repetition rate of between a couple and a few thousand times a second. Electrical appliances, house wiring, TVs, and monitors radiate most at ELF and VLF. Above that in the radio spectrum are LF, MF, and HF, for low, medium, and high frequency. These are used almost exclusively as radio communication bands, and so most computers are shielded at these frequencies to prevent radiation and interference. The same is true of VHF and UHF—very and ultra high frequency—which are used for TV and stereo radio, walkie-talkies, cellphones, and the like. Above UHF is microwave radiation, then comes infrared, visible light, ultraviolet, X-rays, and gamma rays. Although computers radiate some power at all these frequencies, the health effects are well-known and the levels of radiation are kept very low, where appropriate.

How computers emit radiation

Since computers are electrically powered, they must emit radiation of some sort—but how is it different from the negligible and harmless levels of radiation emitted by other domestic and business electrical appliances? As far as the system unit is concerned, it is not. The only source of emissions within the system unit is the power supply, which conforms to the same specification as any other electrically powered apparatus. The real threat comes from the monitor, which contains the control mechanism for displaying screen images.

We have seen how the technology behind a monitor works (see pp. 15-17): An electron gun which receives instructions from the graphics adapter card fires electrons at the phosphor-coated screen, causing the phosphor to glow. This process is harmless; it is the mechanism controlling the movement of the electron gun which represents a potential health hazard. The beam of electrons is accelerated and directed towards the screen by a high voltage transformer, but it requires extra navigational power to move across and down the screen during raster scanning. This is achieved by a horizontal and vertical deflection system: Two sets of coils are wound around the neck of the cathode ray tube and, when the monitor is switched on, electric currents flow through these coils (or yokes) and generate powerful magnetic fields. The magnetic power of these coils is able to deflect the electrons as they are fired from the gun—a horizontal deflection coil moves the beam from left to right; a vertical deflection coil moves it from top to bottom. Each time the electron beam reaches the right-hand side of the screen, a synchronization pulse causes it to "flyback" to the left-hand side while the vertical deflection coil pulls it down a line. Typically, monitors produce 6,262 line pictures a second and the electron beam travels back and forth across the screen more than 15,000 times a second. This amounts to a horizontal scan frequency—or *line refresh rate*—of 15,000 hertz (15 kilohertz); and a vertical scan frequency—or *frame refresh rate* (the entire picture) of 60 hertz.

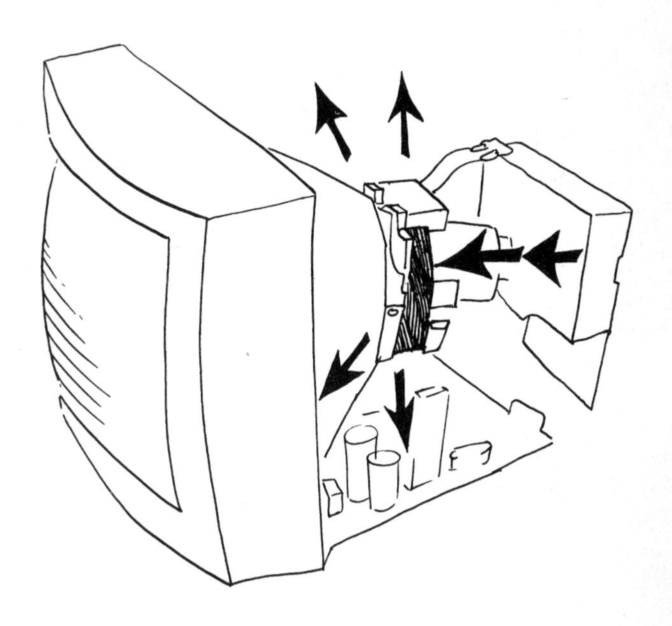

Radiation generated by the deflector yokes is potentially hazardous

This process of image creation in the cathode ray tube gives rise to three types of monitor emissions: X-rays, caused by the impact of the electron beam on the inside of the glass; harmless electrostatic potential, caused by positive voltage on the glass; and alternating electromagnetic fields, caused by the power supply and deflection yokes. The powerful field of electromagnetism generated by the deflector yokes is the source of radiation thought to be harmful to living cells. The monitor is designed to shield the computer user from such radiation: If you look inside a monitor, you will see a lead lining inside the screen which eliminates X-rays almost completely. The glass and casing of the monitor absorb the vast majority of the remaining VLF radiation. Some, however, leaks out—mostly from the back, where the coils are located, some at the side, and a little at the front.

What this means, in physical terms, is that the cyclical movement of the electromagnetic field continues to act beyond the confines of the monitor. An electromagnetic field is composed of charged particles which oscillate (use energy to move back and forth) at a frequency measured in hertz. The frequency at which particles in a particular field oscillate (60 hertz for ELF and 15 kilohertz for VLF radiation) is called the *resonant frequency*, where resonance describes the frequency at which particles will oscillate most freely. All particles (whether in solid, liquid, or gaseous form) have a resonant frequency—what the frequency is depends on the chemical composition of that particle. When a field encounters particles which share its resonant frequency, they too will begin to oscillate at that frequency. The effect is not unlike the movement of a poorly designed suspension bridge: If air currents have been channeled into a particular frequency (by the location of nearby hills, for example) and they hit a suspension bridge, the bridge may begin to move in the same way as the air currents. If the two prove to have the same resonant frequency, the bridge will assume the patterns of oscillation of the air and use its energy to move. The "ripples" of the bridge will continue to increase in size until the whole structure collapses. Humans, like bridges, are also made up of particles which have a resonant frequency. Lest we carry this analogy too far, read the next section for more information about how our bodies interact and respond to different forms of radiation.

The prime suspects: VLF and ELF radiation

VERY LOW FREQUENCY RADIATION

How low-frequency radiation affects cells is still not entirely understood. VLF signals, which range from 3,000 to 30,000 Hz, are emitted primarily by the deflection yokes of monitors and have so far escaped the glare of bad publicity. This does not make monitors entirely innocent: All the recent studies that have given monitors a clean bill of health examined only VLF radiation.

EXTREMELY LOW FREQUENCY RADIATION

Extremely low frequency radiation is at the lowest end of the electromagnetic spectrum. Most physicists define ELF as the radiation band from 30 Hz to 300 Hz, although it is often extended to include any frequency below 30,000 Hz (and therefore VLF). Strictly speaking, ELF is not true radiation, but captive electric and magnetic fields generated by strong electric currents in power systems, appliances, and other electrical equipment (including monitors).

In normal circumstances, we are constantly bathed in very and extremely low frequency radiation, which comes primarily from electricity mains, but also arises naturally from sunshine, fire, hot surfaces, and the earth's own magnetic field. Naturally occurring radiation has no effect on living cells because its resonant frequency is very different from that of the particles found there—this does not seem to be completely true of the artificially generated electromagnetic fields associated with monitors (or electric blankets, hairdryers, and portable telephones, for that matter).

Research into the effects of ELF radiation is increasing, and the phenomenon is now being linked with a variety of health issues. Laboratory studies made on cell cultures and animal tissues, and epidemiological surveys have attempted to find a common link between the backgrounds of sufferers.

Laboratory studies

A large number of laboratory experiments have associated ELF fields with cancer, changes in the biological clock, and subtle alterations to nerve-cell physiology. Research into even mild doses of ELF radiation is beginning to show that, far from being innocuous, ELF electrical and magnetic fields can subtly interact with biological tissue—with both beneficial and harmful effects.

First the good news: ELF fields apparently promote bone growth and hasten healing, and for this reason are commonly used to treat bone fractures. The bad news is that ELF fields also appear to promote the growth of cancerous cells and alter the normal functioning of healthy cells at a very fundamental level. Biophysics suggests that some of the molecules found in living cells, particularly those associated with cell metabolism and cell division, share the resonant frequency of ELF radiation emitted by monitors. If this is the case, the molecules within a living cell would begin to resonate at the same frequency as the particles within a field of ELF radiation when they come into contact with it. If the magnetic fields in this frequency range were biologically active, they could interact with the natural electric activity of the cells, modifying ion balances across cell membranes, growth rates, and nerve-cell behavior. Since such resonance is not normally a part of the cell's activity, its normal life processes would be substantially disrupted.

An interesting effect that laboratory research has turned up is that ELF fields do not behave like high frequency ionizing radiation. ELF fields simply do not have enough energy at the molecular level to change or destroy the chemical bonds in cells; thus, they don't damage chromosomes. Instead, they seem to mimic the electrical changes that normally occur in living cells in the body. By changing the calcium permeability of cells, for example, they can change the response of a nerve cell to stimulation. This can affect a variety of cell functions, including the transmission of electrical signals in nerve tissue.

Matters are complicated by some studies which reveal what is known as the "window effect." Most chemical carcinogens and other types of radiation become increasingly dangerous to living cells as the exposure level increases. Although this is broadly true of ELF, some studies have found that some of the biological effects occur only at certain ELF field strengths (or frequencies) and not at higher or lower values. Furthermore, these window effects appear to depend on the presence and orientation of static field, like the earth's magnetic field. This effect was most clearly demonstrated in one study of chick brain tissue, where cells showed changes in calcium ion levels with 60-Hz ELF fields at field strengths of 35, 40, and 42.5 volts per meter. At field strengths of 25,

30, and 45 volts per meter the same 60-Hz ELF radiation had no effect. The obvious implication of the window effect is that it becomes impossible to develop genuine standards for the emission of electromagnetic radiation. It is made more difficult by the likelihood that the effects of ELF fields would vary with the individual as well, because the size and shape of one's body affects the strength of voltages and currents induced inside it by the ELF fields.

It should be remembered that not all of these reports have been shown to be absolutely true. Other researchers have failed to replicate the results, while still others have found no real link between ELF fields and biological activity. Nonetheless, a consensus is emerging that ELF fields can be biologically active at levels lower than were once thought possible. As a result, many fundamental questions remain unanswered: What constitutes a safe or unsafe level of ELF? Are the effects of exposure cumulative or do they stop when the source is removed? Can sufferers be truly identified—and cured?

Survey findings

A number of epidemiological studies in the late 1980s found abnormally high cancer rates in people living near power lines and using electric blankets, both of which have powerful electrical and magnetic ELF fields. Such studies have generally correlated the illnesses with exposure to ELF fields, although not all have shown a correlation and no link has ever been proven. The results of these studies to date have been mixed. In the United States and Sweden, correlations between cancer and strong ELF fields associated with electrical distribution systems have been found, although contradictory studies have also been published. Taken together, the research findings on ELF radiation do suggest some connection with a number of adverse health effects.

Health issues

Cancer

Cancer is one of the most serious potential side-effects of exposure to ELF radiation, and most of the studies in this area have concentrated on exposure to power lines rather than computers. Research findings in this area seem to suggest that such exposure accelerates the process of cell division, increasing the likelihood of "mistakes" occurring as cells replicate themselves. Furthermore, the rate of increase in cells which are already cancerous is far greater than in normal cells—in other words, exposure to ELF radiation increases the likelihood that a cancer may develop and also encourages the growth of cancers which are already present. Normal immune system defense mechanisms are overwhelmed by this acceleration and cannot cope, allowing malignant growths to develop. As a further complication, studies of rats under ELF exposure point to the suppression of the hormone melatonin as a factor in the development of cancer. Melatonin controls the biological clock, enhances the immune system, and retards the growth of cancer cells. If it is suppressed, of course, the growth of such cells can continue unchecked.

Other theories concentrate on cell membrane activity under the influence of ELF fields. A common resonant frequency and the consequent mimicking of normal cellular processes may be the features of ELF which enable it to contribute to the development of cancer. What appears to happen is that some ELF reactions occur at membrane sites which subsequently exhibit an increased tendency to behave as receptors for cancer-promoting chemicals. In a sort of double negative effect, ELF fields also appear to increase the chemical activity of a compound known as ornithine decarboxylase, a process which has previously been associated with the onset of cancer. The electric field strength of some computer equipment, even at abnormal working distance, appeared near the level at which ornithine decarboxylase activity was found to increase in some studies. In another study, a similar field intensity was found to increase the toxicity of the white blood cells (lymphocytes) which specifically attack cancer cells in mice.

MISCARRIAGE AND PREGNANCY PROBLEMS

The possibility that ELF radiation is connected to pregnancy problems is deeply alarming, and has generated more studies than almost any aspect of computer use. Alarms were first triggered at a newspaper, *The Toronto Star* in Canada, between May 1979 and May 1980. Four women working at the newspaper gave birth to children with different defects—a surprisingly large number—which first led to the association of abnormal pregnancies with monitor use.

A number of American studies took up the banner, rapidly revealing similar statistics across the country. At the Sears Roebuck Company in Dallas, eight out of 12 pregnancies in a year were abnormal and the Attorney General's office in Toronto reported a miscarriage rate of 52 percent over two years. In the Solicitor General's office in Ottawa, seven abnormalities were reported in seven consecutive pregnancies among monitor users.

A rush of research in the mid-1980s failed to find monitors guilty. A Finnish study which drew on the entire country's records of birth malformations failed to find any link between that and monitor use; in Canada and Sweden, two major studies could find no evidence for an association between computer use and any kind of pregnancy problem. A later study, however, did find a link.

In 1988, a carefully controlled study was carried out at the Northern Kaiser Permanente Medical Program, a health maintenance organization in Oakland, California. Researchers, led by Marilyn Goldhaber, followed the lives of 1,583 pregnant women who attended obstetrics and gynecology clinics run by Kaiser, paying particular attention to the environmental hazards these women routinely encountered. Their findings gave cause for concern, expressed by the researchers as a correlation between an increased rate of miscarriages for women who had used VDTs (visual display terminals) for more than 20 hours per week during the first trimester of pregnancy, compared to other working women who reported not using VDTs.

The results are not clear cut, however, with some critics observing that they were not statistically significant. In recognition of this, the researchers themselves drew particular attention to the possibility that women who had adverse pregnancy outcomes may have overestimated their exposure to visual display terminals, while women with normal births may have under-reported theirs. They also acknowledged the role of other factors which the study did not measure, such as poor ergonomic conditions or job-related stress. In the same way that stress plays a role in our susceptibility to repetitive strain injury, it is undoubtedly a factor in the incidence of miscarriage among computer users. One company altruistically offered its pregnant employees lead aprons to wear during computer use, but the practice was abruptly halted after women admitted that wearing the lead aprons was far more stressful than using the monitors.

At least nine subsequent studies have been unable to find a positive association between abnormal pregnancies and monitor usage. In the same year, 1988, also in America, the National Institute of Occupational Safety and Health (NIOSH) studied 882 pregnancies and found that pregnant women who spend a significant amount of time in front of monitors do not run a higher risk of miscarriage. The following year, a study carried out at the University of Toronto showed no association between miscarriages in mice and the electromagnetic fields emitted by computer monitors.

SKIN RASHES

An unusual and rarely reported health condition thought to be linked to electromagnetic radiation is skin rash, usually on the face but sometimes on other parts of the skin. Facial rash was first reported in 1978, almost ten years before the introduction of standards regulating monitor emissions. A team of computer operators working in a factory in London had been using new computers for over a month, when one full-time operator complained of red patches on his cheeks. Two other operators later developed the condition, which then included raised bumps, itchiness, and redness. Similar cases were reported in 1979 in Norway, where operators reported reddish patches, dryness, and tingling of facial skin, which was likened to sunburn. Symptoms appeared up to two hours after beginning work with a computer, and disappeared around two hours after switching it off. An onset was marked by sensations of being patted or stroked with a feather on the affected areas.

Subsequent studies, although few in number, report a consistently higher incidence of skin rash in computer users compared to non-users. In many cases, skin rash occurred in users who had also reported eyestrain and repetitive strain injuries. Fears originally centered around radiation as a cause of skin rash, but research suggests a more indirect relationship. In work locations where several people reported skin rash, researchers also noted new synthetic carpets or recent building work. In both situations, there were abnormally high levels of submicron dust particles in the air. The electrostatic fields generated by monitors have already been shown to attract dust particles by virtue of their opposing charges and this is exacerbated by dryness or low humidity. Where the proportion of dust is high, there will naturally be a higher than normal concentration of particles around a monitor in use. If these particles contain natural irritants—synthetic fibers, brickdust, some chemicals, or even traces of asbestos—the likelihood of an allergic reaction is much higher. In each of these cases, removal of the irritant fibers was associated directly with a decline in reported skin rash. So, although the electrostatic emissions of computers do contribute to skin rash, it is the high concentration of irritant particles drawn to an electrostatic field which actually causes dermatitis.

CATARACTS

In some very rare cases, researchers have found a link between monitor emissions and the development of cataract in some individuals. A cataract is simply an opacity or clouding of the crystalline lens of the eye, leading to a gradual diminution or blurring of vision. Surgical treatment is the only remedy. There are many types of cataract, one of which is associated with radiant energy; ELF radiation from monitors has been implicated in some of these cases. No link has ever been established, since there are many other factors affecting an individual's susceptibility to cataract: Age, medical history, previous injury, and existing visual conditions.

ELECTRICAL HYPERSENSITIVITY

Although monitor emissions have been linked, however tenuously, to damage or irritation of specific parts of the body, it is rare for users to report generalized sensitivity to electricity. In recent years, however, the numbers have been increasing and nearly all the sufferers are habitual computer users. First documented in Sweden in 1987, electrical hypersensitivity is now an identifiable condition with potentially serious consequences.

The first indication that a person is becoming hypersensitive to electricity is minor irritations associated with regular computer use. Typically these include a warm or burning sensation on the face while working with a monitor, and many of the symptoms of skin rash described above. In the hypersensitive, the rash may spread across the body to skin not directly exposed to the monitor. Dryness and irritation of the eyes is common too. In the early stages of hypersensitivity these symptoms fade once the computer is switched off, but they become more persistent and prolonged quite rapidly. The discomfort becomes worse until the facial skin feels as if it is on fire, and other, more alarming symptoms become apparent. These include dizziness, headache, nausea, tooth and jaw pain, aching muscles and joints, and even cardiac palpitations. Other sufferers describe a feeling of impending flu which never quite breaks out.

At first, these symptoms are associated exclusively with computer use but, as they increase in severity, they can be triggered by all sorts of electrical apparatus. Ordinary television sets, fluorescent lights, vacuum cleaners, and electrical cables cause the same reaction, greatly hampering everyday life. In the office, fax machines, pipelines, computer wiring, and liquid crystal clock faces trigger unbearable symptoms. In extreme cases, even daylight, white-painted surfaces, and paper handling can trigger a range of severe and painful symptoms. Electrical hypersensitivity is more than an inconvenience. Extreme cases can be severely debilitating, restricting the sufferer to a life of darkened quiet in an environment free from electrical fields. Work, shopping, and normal life become impossible for the hypersensitive: Interaction with household appliances, electrical cables—even radios—can become unbearable. Inevitably, whole families suffer. Some leave their homes and relocate to remote areas far from electrical activity, where they live by candlelight and cook on wood-burning stoves. Unsurprisingly, many sufferers have to live alone or retreat to mobile homes near the family home.

Sufferers of electrical hypersensitivity react to a far broader range of energy within the electromagnetic spectrum than normal people. Extremely and very low frequency radiation is the first irritant, but symptoms are also triggered by low, medium, and high frequencies (radio waves) and naturally occurring radiation such as infrared and visible light. Swedish research has shown a link between reported feelings of illness and spots of particularly high electromagnetic activity within the homes of people experiencing electrical hypersensitivity; symptoms worsen considerably when, for example, a neighbor switches on a television set next door.

Despite the severity and implications of electrical hypersensitivity, it is not a widely recognized condition. Provocation studies conducted in Sweden in 1993 have been inconclusive: Researchers attempted to provoke the symptoms of electrical hypersensitivity by exposing sufferers to electromagnetic fields. Sometimes the field was switched on and sometimes it wasn't—patients were asked to detect when it was on. Out of thirty hypersensitive subjects who took part, none was able to detect a field with any consistency—successful detections were few enough to have been due to chance alone. Similar studies have had mixed results, with a small number of patients achieving a higher detection rate than can be explained by chance. Others put the condition down to purely psychological factors, having failed to find an objective link between electromagnetism and symptoms of hypersensitivity. Instead, these reports propose a link between the symptoms and the personality of patients—normally hard-working and conscientious but frustrated or under-appreciated.

With little to grasp hold of, tolerance and understanding among Swedish employers (and colleagues) is generally low, yet Sweden is the only country to have put together a formal organization to represent sufferers. The FEB (Foreningen for El-och Bildskarmsskadade, or Swedish Association for the Electrically and VDT injured) has over 1,600 members and claims knowledge of a further 10,000 sufferers throughout Sweden. The condition appears to be peculiar to Sweden, although the FEB cites reports received from many other countries, mainly the Scandinavian countries but also Britain, Germany, Australia, and the United States.

Is electromagnetism harmful or not?

Overall, the evidence implicating computer monitors as a cause of cancer, skin rash, miscarriage, or electrical hypersensitivity is weak, and no scientifically significant results for any such health risks have been reported. Nor should it be forgotten that the difficulties of truly controlling large-scale epidemiological studies are monumental—so many other variables affect the individuals participating that it becomes almost impossible to say with certainty that any one factor is the cause of any one event. All the studies to date are correlational rather than causal, that is, they can show that there is some health effect associated with computer use, but they cannot prove a true cause-and-effect relationship. The radiation from the computer terminals *could* be contributing to health problems, or something else about monitors, or the way a particular study was conducted could have influenced its results.

Most importantly, it is certainly not clear what the specific mechanism is by which electromagnetic radiation could affect a biological process such as pregnancy. The simplest theory proposed a mechanism similar to the theory of accelerated cell division thought to be implicated in the development of cancer. Since fetal tissue is in a state of almost constant and total division, the possibility of errors occurring during uncontrollably accelerated growth is increased enormously, compared with the risk to the cells of a fully grown adult. Such errors are thought to be the triggers of spontaneous miscarriages. The other illnesses discussed here certainly do not require exposure to a computer in order to occur, and the "natural" mechanisms by which they are triggered are no better understood than the computer-related ones. So, although the computer cannot be completely cleared of involvement in health problems, neither can it be unequivocally blamed.

Health factors in the computing environment

WORK SPACE

It should be apparent by now that illness associated with computer use can rarely be attributed to a single cause or factor. More commonly, the complaints that computer users report can be traced back to a vast array of possible sources, from the specifics of a piece of equipment to the vagaries of attitude and environment. It follows, therefore, that our work environment must be one of the possible elements which contribute to our health and well-being (or lack thereof).

Many of the "broader" repetitive strain injuries—head, neck, and shoulder—are the result of more factors than simply fast, repetitive typing. Bad posture, uncomfortable furniture, and a poorly laid out work space all take their toll on the hapless computer user. The work space (also referred to as working environment or workstation) is a rich combination of the following things: The immediate work space comprises personal working habits, the shape and height of the desk, design of the chair, position and angle of monitor, accessibility of the mouse and keyboard, and presence or absence of other items (such as document holders) on the desk. The wider work space also embraces the location of windows, the temperature and humidity of the room, noise, and lighting levels. All these elements contribute to an individual's susceptibility to various health problems. The effects may not be apparent immediately, but the cumulative effects of years spent working on a computer can be damaging.

LIGHTING AND GLARE

Lighting is a surprisingly rich subject of study, both technically and artistically. It also has a profound bearing on our effectiveness as we use computers. There are many terms associated with lighting issues, but the ones of most relevance to visual health are illumination and luminance. *Illumination* is the measure of the stream of light falling on a surface, and its unit of measurement is the lux. Approximately one lux of light is given off by a small candle; a bright, sunny day may reach up to 100,000 lux. Normal office work demands a 100 to 500 lux range, although delicate, detailed work justifies a workplace as bright as 3,500 to 5,000 lux (all of which can be measured by a lighting specialist). *Luminance* is the measure of brightness of a surface—in effect, the amount of light coming from a surface—and is greatly affected by the reflective powers of that surface.

Common Lighting Problems

- Bright walls
- White walls, dark floors
- Reflecting table tops
- Dark office machines on bright tables
- Windows

Many computer users display a preference for dim lighting to achieve better screen contrast. This is fine in itself, but becomes a problem if close paperwork is also required. For most people, the best compromise is reduced overall lighting with an adjustable lamp that can be focused on reading materials but not on the monitor screen. The most painful effect of poor lighting is glare. Glare is caused by the specular reflection of excessive light from the glass surface of the monitor screen. When the eye is trying to focus on information displayed on the screen, the pupil dilates to increase acuity. Glaring light causes the pupil to constrict, however, and the conflict between the pupillary muscle is thought to be the cause of much eye irritation and headache.

Extensive research has been done on the levels of lighting which are appropriate within offices, although the requirements are quite different where computers are used with any regularity. Computer users tend to experience greater contrasts in light and dark, both on the screen and in the surrounding environment, making it important to achieve the optimum balance between screen characters and background (contrast). Extreme contrast, as discussed above, only helps legibility when ambient lighting is carefully controlled, since any extreme luminance from the screen will contrast unpleasantly with the surroundings. Optometrists recommend an illumination level on the desk surface of 300 to 500 lux, which provides the best compromise between lighting sufficient to read paper by, and for comfortable contrast with the monitor. Light much dimmer than this may make the monitor display clearer, but it makes paper much harder to read. It can also have the subtle psychological effect of making users depressed or sleepy. If most of the desk work involves the monitor, it is acceptable to work at the lower end of the recommended illumination level. Lights should be turned up if a high proportion of paperwork is involved.

Guidelines for Light Placement

- No light source in visual field
- Use shades or guards to shield light sources
- Flourescent lights should be aligned directly over work area
- Use power lamps

The source of light is an important part of the overall lighting plan, with direct and indirect sources being typical in an office. Direct light sources send up to 90 percent of their light towards targets in a single cone of concentrated light; indirect light sources, on the other hand, throw the vast proportion of their light onto the walls and ceiling first, from where it is reflected back into the room as a diffuse scattering of light. Direct lighting (e.g., spotlights, focused lamps) is useful as an illuminator of specific areas which need to be clear—faint documents, for example—but it also induces sharply contrasting areas of dark and shade. Indirect lighting achieves a far smoother and more even effect, eliminating glare and shadows. Fluorescent lighting is one of the more harmful sources of direct lighting, since it is composed of flickering light. The flicker is generally a minimum of 100 Hz, which is well above that of most monitors and therefore imperceptible. Nonetheless, it is still within the range of flicker which induces activity within the optic nerve and cannot be ruled out as a contributor to eyestrain. If fluorescent lights are already part of an office layout, flicker can be greatly reduced by using two bulbs together, adjusted to flicker out of phase with one another. This phase-shifting, as it is known, has the effect of turning one bulb on as the other goes off, creating an almost constant light. Phase-shifted fluorescent tubes can be used without any further precautions.

If there is more choice of lighting, one of the most effective ways of ensuring the visual health of computer users is uplighting. The light source should be positioned to point upwards—either directly, or via a shade which deflects light upwards. Uplighters positioned in corners have the added advantage of two opposing walls which further diffuse the light around the room. Where possible, uplighters need to be located at least seven feet above the ground. This ensures that the directed light is still powerful enough to be thrown back evenly by the reflecting surfaces, and it also eliminates the possibility of bright reflections caused by light sources located at head level appearing on monitor screens.

For maximum comfort, the best combination of lighting for the computer is diffuse ambient light, generated by indirect sources and not exceeding 500 lux. If paperwork is a regular part of the job, lighting levels should tend towards 500 lux, or be supplemented by a small, adjustable spotlight for close reading. The aim is to reduce contrast and glare which forces the eyes to work much harder.

TEMPERATURE AND HUMIDITY

The human being is a self-regulating creature, equipped with mechanisms for generating internal stability and responding to external changes. Temperature and humidity are important climatic variables which affect performance at work, particularly in the office environment. Normally, temperature is regulated by internal metabolic processes which conserve or expel heat energy through the dilation or constriction of blood vessels. As body temperature begins to rise, the heart pumps more blood to the cooler surface of the skin where it is dissipated. As this process accelerates, the effect is a reddening of the skin where the local blood vessels dilate to bring more blood to the surface. If blood cooling is not fast enough the skin begins to sweat. As the moisture evaporates, it draws on the heat energy of the skin, cooling it down. In cold climates, the peripheral blood vessels constrict, retaining blood (and hence heat) deep within the body and major organs. Deep body temperature in a healthy person rarely varies by more than a fraction of a degree.

Along with electromagnetic emissions, computers generate heat when they are switched on. Electrostatic charges build up around the screen, aggravated by very dry conditions which allow dust particles to gather in the air. In a large office, the combined effects of heat generation and electrostatic discharge can place a large and expensive load on air conditioning systems. If no such air conditioning exists, employees working in this type of environment quickly become very uncomfortable. Excessive humidity (moisture) in the atmosphere prevents the evaporation of sweat, leaving people feeling stuffy and lethargic. More commonly in a computing environment the problem is excessively dry air, which leaves skin feeling roughened and membranes dry and irritated. The inside of the nose can develop a burning sensation and the eyes often feel red and scratchy. Temperatures much above 76 degrees Fahrenheit have quite marked effects on human performance in the office. The concentration span declines, people performing skilled tasks make more mistakes and may become irritable or lethargic, depending on temperament.

The temperature range at which people are comfortable is surprisingly narrow and very precise, rarely varying by more than two or three degrees from the mean of 74 degrees Fahrenheit. Women tend to prefer a slightly higher temperature than men. Cooling and comfort can be aided by good ventilation, although drafts can be a nuisance. The feet and neck are particularly sensitive to drafts, and most people prefer air currents which come from in front than from behind. Humidity is essential to computerized offices, and most studies recommend relative humidity of 40 to 50 percent, with 30 percent as the absolute minimum. Humidity levels can be "set" in most air conditioning systems; for the home or individual user, it is possible to buy desktop humidifiers. A simple alternative is to place a bowl of water near your desk!

Noise

Noise is an inevitable part of office life, and most of us are able to filter out and ignore sounds which mean little to us. Noise becomes a nuisance when it exceeds levels which we can ignore, even when the content of the sound is irrelevant to what we are doing. Our ability to hear serves primarily as a means of communication between individuals, but it has a secondary role as an alarm mechanism. Unexpected, unfamiliar, or loud noises trigger pathways to the brain which increase alertness and divert mental energy from the task in hand to the interpretation of sound and preparation of an appropriate response. If this happens regularly, it becomes more and more difficult to concentrate. Being in a constant state of mild alarm is also exhausting, making comparatively mild noise levels distracting during office work.

A comfortable level of sound for most people is between 45 and 50 decibels, where the decibel measures the pressure caused by sound waves on the human ear. Computers and computing equipment have introduced new sources and levels of noise to the office environment, some of which exceed this level considerably. Printers are the worst offenders, with matrix and daisy wheel printers producing sound levels of up to 75 decibels, although a hood can reduce this to a more bearable 60 decibels. Computers themselves make almost no noise, although the cooling fan within the system can be clearly heard. At 40 decibels, it is rarely noticed, but some computer cooling fans reach levels of 50 decibels or more. If the office is quiet, or if there is more than one computer, the noise level can become very distracting.

Some computer manufacturers are now going to considerable lengths to reduce the noise levels of their products. Greater insulation within the unit itself reduces noise, and smaller fans are being used. Little can be done to reduce any further the sound of a daisy wheel printer with a hood, although laser printers are almost completely silent.

The use of computerized sound in some offices is becoming a real possibility now, as technological developments continue. Computers have been able to make sounds for many years, but this has rarely been applied to the office environment. The development of sound cards could change this. Sound cards can be slotted into a system unit like a video card, and with the appropriate software, enable a computer to play any type of recorded sound: Music, voices, animal noises, electronic effects—just about anything. This ability has generally been restricted to computer games, but more and more companies are trying to develop serious business applications for computerized sound. It is now possible to control some applications software through the use of sound—instead of selecting "Open" from a drop-down menu to open a new file, or clicking on the word with a mouse, you can simply say "open." Similarly, it is possible to format text by saying "bold," "italic," or "spell." For more complex commands, it is possible to "train" a computer to recognize a specific voice intonation, which increases the accuracy of its understanding. By talking directly to a computer in this manner, it is possible to shave precious seconds off many routine computing tasks.

Sound is being used very effectively by organizations which are geared toward the sight-impaired. It is less easy to foresee an increase of sound cards in open offices, where the cries of "bold," "open," and "quit" would elevate the decibel level way beyond acceptable limits. Not only would the sound be tremendously irritating to those around you, the speakers would also suffer; if not from sore throats, then from the wrath of their colleagues. The question of sound interface is also a serious one: No one would be pleased if a colleague's sudden cry of "Quit" shuts down all the neighboring computers as well as their own; and the use of headphones and microphones is unlikely to be welcome as an alternative since they tend to isolate the listener.

Although computerized sound has some useful specialized applications and interesting potential, it is probably safe to say that, for the moment, it is unlikely to become a significant element of the computer user's office life.

"SICK BUILDING SYNDROME"

Flu-like symptoms in many people in a single office are sometimes ascribed to "sick building syndrome." This combination of lethargy, headache, dry eyes, sore throat, aching muscles, and breathing difficulty seems to occur predominantly in people working in an entirely artificial environment, where the air is conditioned and recycled within a sealed building. The development of symptoms is rarely bacterial in origin, but thought to be due in part to the gradual accumulation of mild irritants such as tobacco smoke, printer emissions, photocopier solvents, and cleaning fluids with little or no fresh air. When combined with a low humidity and high levels of electrostatic charge (from any electrical appliance) the effect can be quite debilitating. Some researchers supplement this research by proposing higher than normal levels of viruses and easier transmission of bacteria in sick buildings, although this has never been supported by medical evidence. The extensive overlap between the sufferers of sick building syndrome and the sufferers of eyestrain and even repetitive strain injury, however, does suggest the influence of broader, stress-related elements at work.

Wider Implications

POWER USAGE AND WASTAGE

Irrespective of the health effects of a single personal computer, the combined effect on the environment of so many computers now in use is substantial. Computers are the leading cause of increased demand for electrical power, accounting for an estimated five percent of commercial demand including industrial and office use, according to one survey. Current estimates predict that the amount of energy soaked up by personal computers could grow by ten percent before the close of the decade. The Environmental Protection Agency studied user habits and discovered that 30 to 40 percent of computer users leave their machines running days, nights, and weekends. Small-scale surveys in Europe indicate a similar proportion there. Reasons given for this practice included impatience with the length of time to boot-up in the morning, use of a remote-control program that requires the base machine always to be on; or an irrational concern that too many power-ons will shorten the life span of vital components. Monitors are a contributor to energy usage too—the same survey estimates that 80 percent of the time a monitor is on, no one is looking at it. So-called screen savers, which purport to prevent phosphor burn when the same image is maintained for hours, actually consume up to 20 percent more energy than a blank screen.

As with all such high energy technologies, the implications are felt at both ends of the process. At the one end, the use of so much electricity contributes to the gradual warming of the atmosphere and widespread "electronic fog" with all its unknown health implications. At the other end of the process, the additional electricity required to generate so much computing power itself requires the extensive consumption of scarce fuels—and increasingly, nuclear energy.

PAPER CONSUMPTION

Computer extravagance is not confined to electricity, however. Despite an earlier, rosier version of the paperless office, computerized offices are using more paper than ever. Not because more people want paper copies of information, but because software and printer technology have led users to expect nothing less than the perfect document. Now, instead of dabbing out minor errors with correcting fluid, users with a boss or clients to impress simply correct the error electronically and print out a new version, sometimes several times. And despite the growth of portable computers, most people still prefer to carry a briefcase of papers to browse through at home or while traveling. It is physically and visually less demanding, if nothing else.

MATERIAL CONSUMPTION

The physical components of computers themselves, and their accessories, represent another potential environmental hazard. Each PC comprises many different materials, many of which are unusable in any other form and cannot be recycled. Desktop and portable machines also rely on batteries for maintenance of their internal clocks—even their entire power supply. If they are the nickel-cadmium type, the main constituent is cadmium, a toxic heavy metal that cannot be disposed of like normal waste. The few recycling programs which exist use the nickel in stainless steel products, although there are plans to replace nickel cadmium batteries with nickel-metal-hydride and eventually lithium cells.

Some of the processes in the manufacture of computer components is environmentally toxic. Semiconductors and hard disks need chlorinated solvents, while processors are etched in microscopic detail with hydrofluoric acid. Like aerosol cans and other producers of chlorofluorocarbons (CFCs), such processes generate long-lived molecules which travel slowly into the upper reaches of the atmosphere, where they can deplete the earth's ozone layer. Publicity generated by aerosol producers has already encouraged computer companies to address this issue, fortunately, and some of the larger, more environmentally-conscientious organizations have switched to a clean "no-wash" manufacturing process that eliminates the use of CFCs.

Printers emit minute quantities of ozone which accumulate in the atmosphere. This gas is implicated in "sick building syndrome" and in the wider issue of air quality generally. Even the toner cartridges within laser printers are of concern, containing highly toxic fluids which cannot be disposed of safely through normal procedures. Some manufacturers of laser printers in the USA offer to recycle used toner cartridges, but only a fraction ever gets returned for subsequent use. Even computer software contributes to environmental damage, as constant upgrades render last month's floppy disks—and their manuals—obsolete. Fortunately, both the plastic and paper used in these elements can be recycled relatively easily, although the burden of responsibility is still very much with users, who can reformat, relabel, and reuse old disks instead of throwing them away. It's also a cheaper way to acquire new blank disks.

Finally, the completed personal computer is lovingly packaged in large quantities of polystyrene and plastic bubble-wrap to cushion its fragile parts from the bumps and shocks inherent in shipping. From cardboard boxes to plastic peanuts, all of this material is discarded after a remarkably short useful life. Enlightened manufacturers have experimented with recycled padding materials and unbleached cardboard boxes. Their experimenting has shown that, on top of the basic savings, compared to white boxes, using brown boxes spares the environment the chemical wastes used in bleaching.

Summary

Working with computers is an interactive process, whereby our mental energy is transferred into electronic output as we type, view, and think. Our interactions are with the computer and with the environment, and the components of office life add up to a dynamic and complex picture.

There have been many suggestions that certain aspects of this interaction are potentially hazardous, and indeed some evidence exists that computerized work places a greater strain on many organs of the human body than paper-based work. It is rarely the entire picture, however. Vulnerability to many of the complaints described in this chapter does not seem to apply evenly to everyone who works with a computer. More powerful predictors of ill-health are complex and hard to quantify, and can rarely be traced to a single cause. There is no question, however, that psychosocial factors are a large element of the jigsaw and remain the most pressing mystery of computer-related health problems.

CHAPTER 5

Computers and Eyestrain

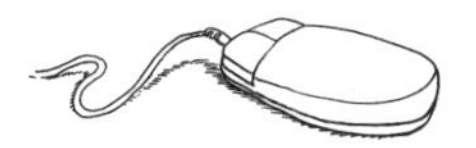

THE EYE IS A COMPLEX and sophisticated piece of machinery, each one nestled deep within the bony sockets of the skull known as the orbits. The eyeball is held in place by six strap-like muscles originated in the back of the orbit which, between them, can move it finely and precisely in almost any direction, around one hundred thousand times a day. Only one-sixth of this delicate device is exposed directly to the outside world, and even this part is carefully protected. The eyebrow and bony brow ridge filter perspiration away from the eye and provide a "bumper" to take the brunt of stray blows. The eyelids and lashes shade and protect the eye and are controlled by reflex mechanisms in the event of unexpected bright lights or rapidly approaching objects.

How the eye works

The eyeball is the part of our body most closely connected to the brain itself. The *retina*, a thin layer of light-sensitive cells which receive and initially process visual input, is actually an extension which grows out from the brain during development of the embryo. Retinal cells have the fastest rate of metabolism in the body, dealing with the synthesis and destruction of visual pigments, the transmission of nerve impulses, and general transport of nutrients. The tough, outer layer of the eye is called the *sclera*, and surrounds the eyeball completely apart from the transparent layer over the pupil and iris. This area is the *cornea*, which partially bends light entering the eye. The lens of the eye is located behind the colored iris and its function is to focus light as it passes the cornea so that it falls exactly on the retina. It does this by expanding and contracting under the influence of the *ciliary muscle*, which alters its curvature to focus light accordingly.

SHORT- AND LONG-SIGHTEDNESS

The closer an object is, the harder the ciliary muscle has to work to squash up the lens and focus its image. Focusing on distant objects allows the ciliary muscle to relax and the lens becomes correspondingly flatter. When the lens is working correctly, light rays are focused to converge exactly on the retina. If the rays converge before they meet the retina, the effect is *myopia* or short-sightedness; a myopic person can only see objects clearly when they are very close—distant objects are just a blur. Myopia is typically a result of the eyeball being a little too long, so that the lens is just behind the point of convergence.

Where the lens causes light rays to converge behind it, the result is *hyperopia* (also known as hypermetropia) or long-sightedness. A long-sighted person can see distant objects clearly but not close ones, often the result of the eyeball being slightly too small. As people age, they tend to become slightly long-sighted; this is because the lens loses its elasticity and it becomes progressively more difficult for the ciliary muscles to adjust. This condition, known as *presbyopia*, can actually reduce the severity of some cases of myopia.

The causes of short- and long-sightedness (known jointly as *refractive error*) are not thoroughly understood, but are thought to be largely genetic in origin. Myopia generally begins at an early age and is fully developed by the early twenties, and little can be done to reverse this process. The rarer, later onset of myopia occurs after that age, and seems to be more closely associated with visual work. Highly literate cultures tend to have a higher proportion of myopics than illiterate cultures, suggesting that regular, close reading work does have an effect on the development of myopia. (A more sinister observation on the significance of myopia is the policy of the Khmer Rouge in Cambodia, who began their extermination of the intelligentsia in the 1960s by targeting the wearers of spectacles.)

COLOR VISION

Human beings are one of the relatively few species able to detect color. This is made possible by the presence of microscopic cone-shaped cells in the eyeballs which are tuned to detect different wavelengths of light, exclusively red, green, and blue. The cones, as they are known, are concentrated around the back and center of the eyeball where the optic nerve leaves the eyeball. Other areas of the eye are more richly populated with rod-shaped cells (the rods) which can distinguish only between dark and light. Because they are distributed more densely farther away from the optic nerve, it can be easier to see objects in dim light by looking just slightly away from them rather than directly at them.

Color blindness is a peculiar defect of the cones, the most common being an inability to distinguish between red and green. This happens because the cones produce abnormal pigments, but the cause is actually genetic, linked to gender. There are variations of color blindness, although complete color blindness—monochromatic vision—is extremely rare.

How computers affect the eye

Computer use requires that a considerable length of time, in some cases several hours, be spent staring at the screen of a monitor. This practice has given rise to an increase in levels of reported general eyestrain, and some researchers even believe there is a link between extensive computer use and cataract. Awareness of visual ergonomics can be used to limit eyestrain experienced as a result of computer usage.

Symptoms of general eyestrain or visual fatigue include soreness, redness, a dry or gritty sensation in the eyes, inflammation of the eyelids and surrounding membranes, difficulty in focusing, blurred or double vision, dizziness, nausea, and headache. The symptoms arise from overuse of the muscles in and around the eye, particularly the orbital muscles which control movement of the entire eyeball, and those used for adjusting the lens during focusing. Frowning, clenching the jaw, and holding the head in a static posture all contribute to these symptoms.

Over the past ten years, a number of researchers have surveyed computer users to assess the scale of reported eye problems. Results have varied from as few as 25 percent of the survey populations to as many as 85 percent complaining of visual difficulties, but substantial methodological differences make it difficult to compare these studies with any certainty. Nonetheless, eye professionals agree that computer-related eyestrain is typically short-lived and reversible. There is nothing in the above research to suggest that even prolonged monitor use contributes to the development of true, permanent myopia, or short-sightedness.

Studies conducted over five years in Canada and two-and-a-half years in Holland found no deterioration in vision from computer use that could not be attributed to normal aging. Based on this and other extensive studies, the American Academy of Ophthalmology in 1984 concluded that existing evidence indicated that monitors were safe for normal use and presented no hazard to vision.

Myopic or not, many people find the symptoms of eyestrain a significant problem which occurs predominantly in conjunction with computer use. In a 1988 study, 26 percent of the participants developed significant temporary myopia after computer usage, and another 42 percent showed changes bordering on significant. A 1984 study showed that after working on a VDT, the time required to shift focus between near and far objects increased, and a 1981 study showed an increased incidence of eye fatigue and irritation among computer users compared with other office workers, although eye examination showed the same level of eye problems in both groups.

Broader and narrower studies have since sought the cause of these irritations, and most research points in one direction. Eyestrain seems to be not a function of computers themselves but of how, where, and under what conditions they are used. Ergonomic reviews attribute eye irritations to factors such as glare, improper lighting, improperly corrected vision, and poor arrangement of work materials, although there are specific features of monitor set-up which can contribute to the symptoms of eyestrain. In total, eyestrain is a result of four broadly defined factors: The monitor, the workstation, work practices, and individual differences, especially existing (uncorrected) eye defects.

THE MONITOR

Radiation

As we saw in Chapter 4, extremely low frequency (ELF) radiation, emitted by the monitor's deflection coil, is thought by some researchers to play a part in some biological abnormalities including cancer, skin rashes, and miscarriage. Ophthalmologists believe ELF to be the most likely factor in a certain type of cataract known to be caused by radiant energy, although there is no evidence that the emissions of monitors are in any way linked to (the very rare) cases of this condition.

Electrostatic fields

An electrostatic field is composed of charged, stationary particles which build up as the electron gun fires electrons at the back of the screen. Although harmless in themselves, negatively charged electrostatic particles attract positively charged particles, including dust, which can cause irritation to eyes and sometimes skin. The extent and severity of irritation, however, is far more dependent on the nature of the dust particles than the way they are attracted toward the monitor.

Flicker

Screen flicker is caused by the sweeping action of the electron gun as it refreshes the screen image. On most monitors this happens between approximately 60 and 70 times a second, where it is imperceptible when stared at directly. If the screen refresh rate is less than 60 times a second, or if it is perceived peripherally, it is possible to detect flicker which can be intensely irritating to the eye. Optical research suggests that although people cannot observe flicker at 70 Hz or above, there is sufficient activity in retinal cells and along the optic nerve to suggest that flicker is nonetheless perceived. Startling studies have shown activity of this kind at refresh rates of 120 Hz—nearly double the accepted standards. What this means, in effect, is that text displayed on a screen is a complex combination of spatial and temporal modulation and is physically very different from information printed on paper.

The perception of flicker is also a major factor in the development of visual fatigue. When reading paper-based text, the part of the brain which processes visual input (the visual cortex) works in small bursts of rest and activity. These bursts correspond to signals received from the eye as it distinguishes between meaningful information (text) and black background (paper). When the eye gazes at a monitor, it does not perceive the non-text area as blank; instead, it perceives flicker. Since this is registered as some sort of information (albeit different from the text), the brain must process it, losing its moments of rest as it does so. The visual cortex is therefore working constantly during computer use, whereas in normal circumstances it maintains a series of pauses during reading. Reading a computer display is literally harder work than reading a sheet of paper.

Color

Colors which lie at opposite ends of the spectrum require the eye to adopt different degrees of focus. It is important, therefore, to avoid color schemes which put, for example, red and blue together. Otherwise, color preference is largely a matter of personal taste, in which case the ability to configure color schemes is more important than the availability of any particular set of colors. Color is critical only where users suffer from impaired color vision—one in eight men is estimated to suffer from some form of color blindness, the most common being an inability to distinguish between red and green.

These factors all have some bearing on reported eyestrain, although it is unlikely that they are significant. The quality of monitors has improved tremendously in recent years, bringing higher resolution, reduced flicker, and minimal electrostatic levels to the desks of most users. For this reason, studies of eyestrain have broadened the field of research to look at the complete workstation.

THE WORKSTATION

The term "workstation" is usually taken to mean the immediate working environment of the computer user: System unit, monitor, and keyboard, as well as desk, chair, and lighting. Several components of the workstation have implications for visual health.

Angle and position

The location of the monitor in relation to its operator has an important bearing on visual health. The normal viewing angle of the eye is approximately 15 degrees below the horizontal plane—in other words, people prefer to look down slightly rather than directly ahead to read something. This angle should be maintained when viewing the display on a monitor, for two reasons. Primarily, when you are gazing directly ahead at something, the eyes are open much wider than is comfortable for prolonged periods. The eyelid is drawn back, exposing more of the cornea to air currents and dust particles and increasing the chances of soreness, dryness, and irritation. The second reason is that gazing directly ahead holds the head and neck at a slightly unnatural angle, tilting the head too far back and imposing extra load on the neck. This creates tension in the neck muscles which can generate persistent headaches and, quite often, a sensation of pain or burning deep behind the eyes.

Viewing distance

Most people remember being told, at some time in their childhood, not to sit so close to the television. Being close up to an image does increase the focusing effort the eye has to make, increasing the rate at which fatigue develops. It is not clear whether it also increases the likelihood of short-sightedness developing—most optometrists think not—but it can bring on other symptoms such as headache and neck tension. Normal reading distance is about 18 inches whereas most monitors are positioned at around 21 inches from the operator. This is a good thing, reducing the strain the eye is under, but it does have implications for older users. As the eye ages, it loses its ability to change focus from a near to a distant object, such that most people require reading glasses by the age of 45. If the lenses are adjusted to a normal reading distance of 18 inches, the screen will not be clearly focused; if they are adjusted to the screen, paper-based reading will be more difficult.

Lighting

Lighting is a complex subject, discussed in more depth below. It does, however, have a specific role to play in relation to the monitor and vision independently of the working environment. The factor that makes the viewing of a monitor different from the viewing of paper in the same lighting conditions is that monitors themselves emit light. Although the eye is equally able to deal with emitted or reflected light, this difference affects the optimum lighting requirements for each situation.

When light falls on a monitor screen, it hits first the polished glass surface of the screen, and then the roughened phosphor coating on the back surface. Light which is reflected by the glass will form a precise, clear reflection of the light source—a window or lamp, for example, This is called a *specular reflection*. Because of the screen's curvature, the reflected image will be smaller than its source and slightly curved. Light reflected by the roughened phosphor, on the other hand, will go in all directions, giving an effect of diffuse light radiating from the monitor at all times. With no ambient lighting (a darkened room) the contrast between dark text and a light background is at its greatest, creating a highly legible image. The contrast between the display and surrounding environment is too great, however, forcing the eye to readjust continually to the bright monitor and then the dark room. If, on the other hand, a light source is shone directly at the monitor, not only is there an increase in obtrusive specular reflections, but the contrast on the display is greatly diminished.

WORK PRACTICES

Staring at anything for hours at a time is tiring to the eyes, and a relatively unusual activity. Paper-based reading induces eyestrain in exactly the same way as gazing at a monitor does—both activities fatigue the muscles of the eye the way that any sort of physical exertion fatigues the muscles involved. This is further aggravated if a user develops the habit of frequent head-turning, to focus on paper and monitor alternatively. Eliminating all the factors discussed above will not, therefore, eliminate eye fatigue if users continue to gaze at the monitor for extended periods. Certain work practices encourage users to remain at their desks and carry on working: They may be paid on a keystroke per hour rate, for example. This is unhealthy and counterproductive—such practices are also widely incriminated in the development of repetitive strain injuries.

Individual Differences

EYE DEFECTS

No amount of adjustment to the monitor or workstation will prevent eyestrain in individuals whose eyes are already defective. If defects have been identified and corrective measures implemented, that person is neither more nor less vulnerable to eyestrain than the next, but undetected defects will make monitor usage far more difficult. Other, minor deficiencies which are not noticeable in everyday situations may become more apparent and more problematic in the tiring visual environment of the computer. Monitor viewing places heavy demands on the visual system, requiring sustained focusing, frequent eye movements, precise visuo-motor coordination (especially when using a mouse or other pointing device) as well as sustained concentration. It is far more likely that, in these circumstances, a person will become aware of existing defects such as poor ocular coordination or local nerve supplies. For these reasons, a regular eye test is important.

BLINK RATE

Studies show that when people are staring at a monitor and concentrating on a task, blink rate drops dramatically. This reduces the rate at which the lachrymal (tear) glands rinse the surface of the eye, causing dryness, grittiness, and increased vulnerability to dust particles. The simplest way to overcome this is to force yourself to maintain a frequent blink rate—think about blinking and make a conscious effort to do it more often while using a computer.

PSYCHOLOGICAL FACTORS

As with many of the computer-related ailments discussed in this book, reported eyestrain is subject to the influence of a wide range of psychological factors. Like the victims of RSI, sufferers of eyestrain are often those people whose job satisfaction actually falls following the introduction of computer power. The link is direct in many ways: Jobs which were previously diverse are now far more restricted, requiring employees to perform a far larger proportion of their work in front of a monitor. This leads directly to higher rates of eye fatigue, headache, and irritation. With less need to move around and interact, however, some employees find their work far more isolated once a computer is introduced. New skills are required, quite often to achieve fewer goals, and the work may be generally less enjoyable. Generalized discontent of this kind may make users more aware of and more likely to report minor symptoms.

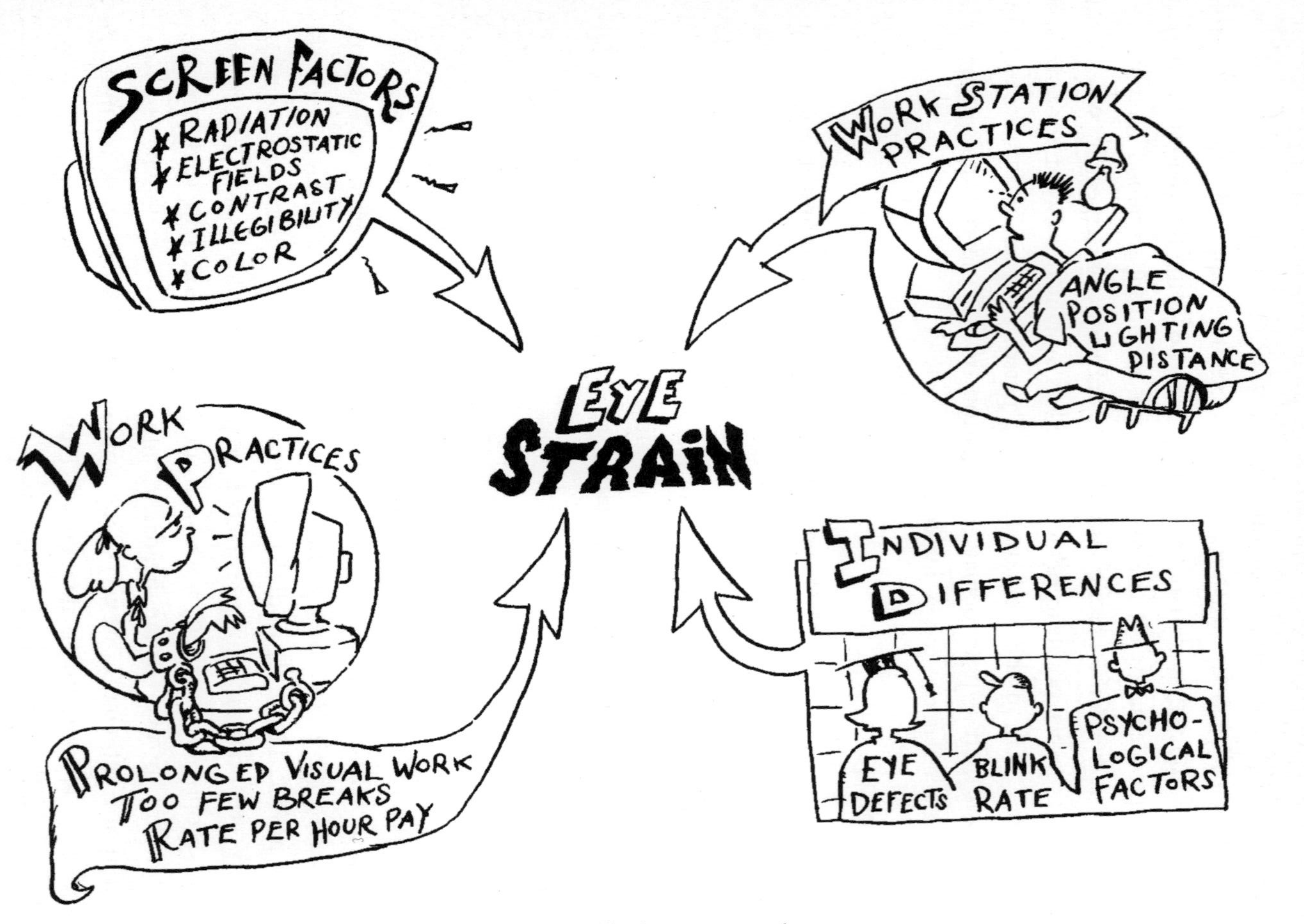

Factors contributing to eyestrain.

CHAPTER 6

Preventing and Treating Computer-Related Health Problems

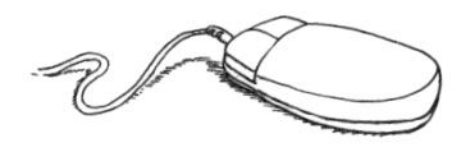

THE RANGE OF TREATMENTS FOR computer-related injury is small but diverse and growing all the time. Most professionals who treat RSI, eye-strain, rashes, and other problems agree, however, that the earlier a cure can be applied the greater the chance of a complete recovery. The chances of continued good health are greatest when injuries are prevented from even beginning.

Prevention: Stop problems before they start

Without a doubt, the prevention of the complex and poorly understood health complaints associated with computer use is the best way to tackle them. Since many of the complaints appear to be cumulative rather than sudden, any delay in treating early symptoms is damage. Prevention begins with understanding how and why they start, and taking measures to avoid or minimize the habits, equipment, and environmental factors which are implicated in computer-related injury.

Good habits

"It's not what you do, it's the way that you do it" applies as accurately to computing as to any other life endeavor, so don't blame your personal computer, look at the way you use it. Whether people are working in an office or at home, the way they learn (or choose) to interact with their computers influences their state of physical and mental health. Explaining and encouraging good usage habits from the first opportunity, whether through training or personal interest, will save a fortune in subsequent health care bills. The most constructive practices are simple to learn and cheap to implement too.

CONTROL AND RESPONSIBILITY

Good computer relations start with a sense of personal responsibility for the work going on inside the box as well as for the wider working environment. Encouraging a sense of ownership in people for the work they do means they have more of themselves invested in the end product—and fewer reasons to feel bored or underutilized. The same is true of their involvement in the choice of machinery, furniture, and software—the earlier people can be involved in the buying process, the less reason they will ultimately have for complaint. People care more when they have personal interests at stake: If employees are allowed to define their personal working space, they develop a sense of ownership and responsibility for the entire job.

Pride in the workplace and what goes on there can be maintained by routine environmental maintenance—in other words, tidying your desk. A surprising amount can be achieved by carrying out this humble task, even for those creative types who swear their messy desks reflect their energetic minds. Organizing pens and clearing in-trays of the paraphernalia of completed projects, returned phone calls, used research, and out-of-date memos can be very therapeutic. It provides a physical break from the immobility and tension of prolonged computer use and frees valuable space for the optimum positioning of monitor, keyboard, and peripherals. It also helps to clear the mind and focus mental resources on what still needs to be done, rather than letting it dwell on what you might or might not have finished. It will probably also turn up that paperwork that you can't get along without, but thought you were never going to see again.

Employers should steer clear of incentives (or pressures) which encourage more rapid data entry. Measuring the performance and wages of data input staff in terms of keystrokes per hour is the quickest shortcut to more errors, more RSI, and more litigation. It applies an unbearable pressure on people who may not have had the necessary keyboard training, eliminates any feeling of control or responsibility they may have had, and ultimately cripples productivity. It is far more constructive to specify a target for the day or even the week, and then let staff schedule their own time to take breaks and meet targets.

MICROPAUSES

A growing body of research is highlighting the importance of short breaks, or micropauses, in the prevention of computer-related health complaints. The term means what it says—tiny breaks (in terms of time) can provide much-needed rest and recuperation for tired muscles and eyes. A typical micropause might be no more than a glance away from the screen, the stretching and flexing of the arms, and a brief rotation of the head and neck. If practiced regularly, micropauses can keep you going for hours. Ergonomists and other specialists recommend thirty-second micropauses every five to ten minutes, with a longer pause (ten to fifteen minutes) after every hour of continuous working. This would normally involve moving away from the computer—perhaps to make a cup of coffee or file some papers. Depending on the nature of the work, longer breaks need to be taken every three to five hours—an hour for a meal, a long walk, or another entirely different activity. Scheduled and practiced regularly, there is powerful evidence that micropauses keep computer users happier, healthier, and more productive in the long and short term.

Adjustable equipment

The equipment you use can say a lot about your budget, but only the way you choose and use the overall combination of personal computer, peripherals, and immediate working environment can make a difference to your health. The watchword for all preventative equipment and furniture is *adjustability*—don't expect to buy perfect equipment, expect to buy adjustable equipment which can be made perfect in different ways for everyone who needs to use it.

MONITORS

These should be angled away from direct light sources to minimize glare, a solution which is cheaper and frequently more effective than anti-glare screens. They should be positioned so that users look down at them at an angle of around 15 degrees, maintaining a distance of about 30 inches between face and screen. It is tempting to save desk space by placing the monitor on top of the system unit but, if the desk is the correct height, this will raise the monitor above a comfortable viewing location. Often the best solution to problems of space and convenience is to locate the system unit beneath the desk, either hooked directly beneath its surface or held upright in a floor bracket. All monitors are now required by law to be of the "tilt and swivel" variety, such that they rest on a base which allows them to be tilted up or down and swiveled from left to right. This adjustability is essential for eye and neck health and, when applied correctly, can greatly reduce the incidence of neck pain and headache.

Controlling monitor emissions

The position and location of the monitor is a relatively simple problem to tackle, compared to the issue of emissions and electrical hypersensitivity. If it is accepted that monitor emissions do occur, even if it is still unclear how damaging they are, there are steps that can be taken to reduce or even eliminate the types and levels of emission.

Reducing electrostatic potential

Most manufacturers now incorporate a simple grounding device within their monitors which almost entirely eliminates electrostatic potential. A thin conducting film is laid across or within the glass screen of the monitor, which is then connected to the chassis ground of the monitor. Happily, no further steps need to be taken by the user. Monitors which do not have a grounding device will retain high levels of electrostatic potential which, although harmless in itself, attracts dust and particles which can be irritating to skin and eyes. Although it is difficult to reduce electrostatic charge, it is possible to control its effects by keeping the monitor, its screen, and the surrounding environment as clean as possible. It is possible to buy monitor cleaning spraysor wipes which dampen electrostatic levels temporarily, and regular dusting or wiping will minimize the level of dust in the air (as well as maintaining a crystal-clear image on the screen).

Reducing electromagnetic fields

Whatever the true effect of electromagnetic radiation (if any), most manufacturers have sensibly taken the stance that addressing the issue is preferable to ignoring it. The difficulty has been to strike a responsible balance between educating and protecting the user population, and simply scaremongering. A controversial advertisement for low-emission monitors, depicting the fetus and implying that its health was at risk if its mother worked with an ordinary monitor, was withdrawn almost immediately following anxious inquiries from users and employers and condemnation from the scientific community. Since then, most manufacturers have chosen to comply with standards which specify emission levels felt to be well below safe levels for human users. These standards have been developed over a period of years on the basis of extensive research into physics and cell biology.

Actual techniques to reduce emission levels are relatively simple and need not add much to the cost of a monitor. At its simplest, reduced emissions are achieved by using a smaller "cancellation coil" to counteract the main deflection coil's magnetic field. The two fields oppose each other, canceling each other out and generating lower emissions. Other techniques include the use of anti-static and anti-glare coatings within the monitor tube; and more extensive shielding of the monitor housing to prevent electromagnetic fields from escaping at the back and sides of the monitor. New display technologies eliminate emissions altogether, such as the liquid crystal displays discussed in more detail in Chapter 2. At the time of writing, these flat panel displays are extremely expensive and mostly restricted to high quality notebook computers—it is to be hoped that their availability and applicability will increase with time, especially as awareness of their health benefits grows among users.

One American manufacturer has developed a keyboard which incorporates its own small electromagnetic coil which is switched on when the computer is in use. The Keytronic keyboard works on the same principle as the cancellation coil within the monitor, generating its own electromagnetic field which disrupts that being emitted from the monitor (and is likewise disrupted by the monitor's field). Exactly how effective it is at dispersing "harmful" radiation is unclear—what is certain is that it is not going to make it any worse.

KEYBOARDS

Current ergonomic expertise recommends keyboards of no more than 1¼ inch thickness (at the middle) with the keys measuring somewhere between ½-¾ inch square. The angle of incline should be between 10 and 15 degrees, and adjustable via legs on the lower surface. Keying action is often a matter of personal preference, but it is important that each depression should provide some form of feedback, such as a clicking noise or feel. To understand keyboard technology better, refer back to Chapter 2. Keyboards must also be detachable from the main computer. This goes without saying for desktop personal computers, but notebooks are a loophole. It is not advisable to use or let employees use notebooks as their main desktop machine—desirable as they are, they are not designed for prolonged use and will exacerbate musculoskeletal problems. New legislation makes a detachable keyboard compulsory, so notebook users who cannot be parted from their portables will have to plug them into a separate monitor if the notebook is their main machine.

Of all the components that have received the attention of designers and ergonomists, the keyboard has perhaps changed the least. Monitors and system units have been redeveloped extensively but, despite the best attempts of researchers, the keyboard has remained stubbornly the same. The commercial manual typewriter was introduced in 1874, followed by the electric typewriter in 1934. Back in the nineteenth century, the keyboard skills of typists frequently exceeded the capabilities of the machine and so a typewriter designer, Charles Sholes, redesigned the layout. The result of his work was the original QWERTY keyboard layout—*specifically intended to slow typists down*, thus avoiding the frequent key jams that plagued them in those early days. Nor is the QWERTY layout random: The choice of key placement was the result of a letter combination frequency analysis. Letters that were frequently adjacent to one another in words were moved to opposite ends of the keyboard, preventing successive keys from jamming each other as they arose from the arc of the key bed resting site to meet at the platen.

Of course, the justification for the QWERTY layout disappeared with the arrival of the electronic typewriter, but by then a whole generation of typists had learned the awkward layout. Suggestions for a rearrangement of the keyboard are certainly not new, and a wealth of studies exists to prove that the QWERTY layout requires the typist to assume postures of the trunk, head, shoulders, arms, and hands that are "unnatural, uncomfortable, and fatiguing." The reason for this is the distribution of the workload across each hand. Ideally, the layout of keys should be determined by the relative strength of each finger and the frequency with which certain letters occur in a certain combination. The QWERTY keyboard allocates most of the typing workload to the left hand, reflected in some studies which record a slightly higher incidence of repetitive strain injuries on the left side of typists. Only a third of keystrokes are allocated to the home keys (those at the typist's fingertips when resting), putting additional load on the weaker, outer fingers and forcing typists to bridge large gaps when typing commonly occurring letters.

Concern with the deliberately poor design of the QWERTY layout led Alphonse Dvorak, as far back as 1936, to investigate an alternative. Using the same principles which were applied to make the QWERTY layout slow and inconvenient, Dvorak developed the *Dvorak keyboard* layout, placing the keys for maximum convenience and efficiency. This layout redistributes more of the workload to the right hand and over two-thirds of all keystrokes to the home keys. Although eminently more sensible than the QWERTY layout, the Dvorak alternative has never become widely used.

More recent studies of keyboard use have focused particularly on detailed physiological considerations of a worker at the keyboard. Klockenberg, who used this research to propose the *Klockenberg split keyboard* layout alternative, offered a number of still valid suggestions. One was to tilt the keyboard sections allotted to each hand concurrently to the left and right sides, respectively, in order to alleviate muscle tension in the typist's shoulders and arms by reducing the angles at which the forearm and wrist are flexed. Other observations led to the formulation of some basic principles or objectives upon which to create the skeleton of new keyboards, these being reduced finger travel during typing and a more natural posture and movement pattern for keying. This idea is further developed in the two-handed *Maltron Ergonomic split keyboard*, designed in the United Kingdom by Stephen Hobday. It divides the alphabet keys into two groups and places them in hemispherical indentations on either side of the case. The functions keys line the top while the numerics are arranged in typical fashion in the center of the keyboard. Shift, Enter, Ctrl, Alt, End, Home, and cursor keys are placed in mini-indentations near the lower corners of the alphabet keys—about where your thumbs would be as you were typing. The Maltron offers the standard QWERTY layout as well as its own ergonomic layout, designed using similar principles to those underlying the Dvorak layout. A single key will switch it from one layout to another, but to use the Maltron layout permanently you have to buy a different set of key caps to indicate which letter is which.

The increasing range of different circumstances in which people find themselves using computers has led to a number of quite radical keyboard alternatives. *Chord keyboards* enable a user to type ostensibly much faster, but he or she must first learn combinations of keys to type different characters—rather like making different notes on a piano. One design uses only half the keys of a normal keyboard but allocates two characters to each. An additional key switches between the two sets, enabling users to type with just one hand, switching when necessary to gain access to the full range of characters.

It seems strange that, despite the problems of the QWERTY layout and the availability of so many more appropriate alternatives, none of these has gained anything more than a tiny share of the keyboard market. The most likely reason is simply that generations of typists have invested too many long and painful hours learning the QWERTY layout and are not prepared to put in similar effort for a different layout. Until this happens, no manufacturer will be able to sell an alternative keyboard in large quantities, thus creating a Catch-22 situation of supply and demand. Any attempt to revise the current key layout pattern radically and irrevocably will face an insurmountable obstacle. An unfamiliar key arrangement would require millions of individuals to relearn typing skills, requiring extensive training and a large bill to employers for the replacement of current keyboard equipment.

As is the case for so many designs, the real key to success and maximum acceptance is flexibility. A natural posture for keying to maximize comfort requires that the keyboard be freely adjustable to the individual typist's natural posture. Each person is different to some degree, either slightly because of physical dimensions or more so due to physical disabilities or handicaps. Ideally, then, one could argue that the ideal keyboard should have separately and independently adjustable sections so that the loads of left and right hand could be set according to individual preference. This might vary, for example, depending on the hand of preference of the typist, the language or dialect being used and even the nature of the work being typed. Highly technical or scientific articles, for example, would make greater use of the keypad and extended character set for scientific and mathematical notations. It seems likely that the progress of technology will make programmable keyboards of this nature available before too long.

Pointing Devices

Of these keyboard alternatives, by far the most popular is the mouse. The pointing device was a revolutionary concept when first introduced, offering a truly radical alternative to the keyboard. It was developed as an accompaniment to the icon-based graphical user interface (GUI), described in Chapter 2, and was intended to enable users to simulate the effect of pointing at an item in order to indicate its selection. For this reason, pointing devices are meaningless when used in a non-graphical (or character-based) interface except where the elements of the GUI are incorporated—such as drop-down menus or dialog boxes. Pointing devices have become widely accepted by users of the GUI, although they are unlikely ever to replace the keyboard. Proficient users of the keyboard still assert that familiar combinations of two or three keystrokes are quicker than a mouse when executing certain commands, and touch-typists find it positively disruptive to leave their keyboards and handle a mouse. Pointers are useful for beginners, and during the launch and administration of an application, but the real meat of information processing remains the province of the keyboard. Nonetheless, the pointing device is a focus of intensive human-computer interaction and has attracted considerable attention for its role as a factor in the development or prevention of musculoskeletal aches and pains.

The basic mouse best encapsulates the purpose and concept of the pointing device—a remote tool, sensitive to the movements of hand and finger, whose movements are duplicated on the screen with an appropriate gradation of fineness. The use of two buttons on the right- and left-hand sides controlled by the forefinger and middle finger, respectively (pointing, single and double clicking with the right- and left-hand buttons), adds a new level of complexity to the range of commands made available with a mouse. In combination with the software (which must be designed to be sensitive to the actions of the mouse), users can now apply different clicks to select single characters, strings of characters (words), sentences, or paragraphs. By holding one button down, they can either execute a selected command or literally *drag* a selected item across the screen and *drop* it somewhere else. The concept of "drag and drop" has become one of the most useful and effective attributes of the mouse.

Because of its popularity, the mouse has been the object of much redesign by ergonomists, with varying degrees of success. The best efforts to design a mouse which prevents injury have attempted to take account of the shape and position of the human hand during mouse usage. Typically, the hand is curved over the mouse, with the thumb and little finger resting on the sides, and the fore and middle fingers poised over the buttons. Good designs incorporate a similarly curved shape such that the palm of the hand is fully supported and the fingers do not need to stretch too far to reach the buttons. The buttons themselves have to be sufficiently sensitive to respond to quite gentle pressure, but not so sensitive that they can be triggered accidentally by a resting digit. Sometimes the left button is larger than the right since it is more frequently used by the forefinger, although this causes problems for left-handers who have switched the function of the buttons. In fact, this type of overdesign is a problem for the mouse in general. One model includes grooves in the shape and position of the fingers, as if a hand had squeezed a large block of soft clay and left finger indentations. Although marvelously comfortable for people with exactly that hand shape, this mouse is quite unusable for anyone with hands smaller than those used to create the original model—most women, in effect.

Other forms of pointing device include the *graphics tablet* (generally restricted to specialized drawing applications); the *trackball*, a sort of upside-down mouse where the cursor is controlled by the thumb; and a range of electronic pen-like devices which mimic the shape and appearance of a normal pen. Despite the range of alternatives and the impressive ergonomic theory behind them, few pointing devices besides the mouse have really caught on. Some have been deliberately restricted to specialized users, although others lack certain fundamental ergonomic principles. The trackball, for example, tends to rely heavily on the thumb or forefinger to control its gross movements, leaving precision control of the buttons to the less sensitive middle finger. If this is not successful, the forefinger must perform this task in addition to controlling the ball, meaning that it must jump from ball to button at intervals, which is rarely satisfactory. *Pen mice*, shaped like a pen, enable a user to hold the pointer in a familiar and comfortable position, but rarely seem to consider that the users of real pens do not have to control two further buttons. Pen mice also require an electronically sensitive pad on which to write, to be sure that commands are transmitted from the point to the screen. Selection of items may be done either by pressing the point of the pen hard against its mat, or by clicking buttons located on the side of the device. Neither of these actions represents the normal and comfortable use of a pen. As such, the pen mouse is a good example of a poorly executed metaphor (also discussed in Chapter 2), resembling an everyday object in appearance but failing to extend the metaphor to its actions. That said, there are people who have become used to the pen mouse and swear by it as the best type of pointer. The same could be said of any product which requires time and effort to be invested in learning it.

Only as part of the portable notebook computer has the mouse been developed with true ingenuity. Since mice with long extension cables and mats are clearly impractical on a notebook, a range of built-in devices have been developed to replace them. The most common is the familiar trackball, first introduced to the notebook by Apple and now widely adopted throughout the industry. A Microsoft design, separate from the main machine, slots onto the side of the notebook, while others are located above and below the main keyboard. The thumb controls the ball and the buttons are generally to the left and right of it, although the best designs curve the buttons or locate them more directly beneath the fore and middle fingertips, as they would be positioned in relation to the thumb. A particularly clever design by Compaq put the trackball on the bottom right-hand corner of the inside of the notebook lid, with the two buttons directly opposite on the outside. Thus, when the lid was flipped up as in normal use, the user could control the ball with the thumb while the fore and middle fingers rested naturally and comfortably on the right- and left-hand buttons respectively. Another notebook alternative is IBM's tiny *track point*, a rubber-coated button the size and shape of a lentil or small bean, which lies somewhere between the two home keys, F and J, on the keyboard.

It works something like a joystick, such that pressure on it from the fingertip moves the cursor in the same direction, although the track point itself remains stationary. The buttons are located elsewhere, normally below the keyboard to allow access during track point use. Some users report that the track point is the most accurate pointing device, although most agree that it has not solved the problem of button location as effectively as the lid-located trackball design.

The biggest problem with many notebook pointing devices is that they tend to be designed for the right-handed user only. Since designers have intentionally eliminated cords, cables, and mats, it is impossible for left-handed users to adapt these devices for their own use, and must therefore adapt their left-handedness instead. The alternative is compromise, where the trackball is located in the center of the machine and can be used by both left- and right-handers, although the location is ideal for neither. The track point is the least hand-biased pointer and is being adopted by some manufacturers as a permanent feature of the keyboard, whether for notebook or desktop machines.

ERGONOMIC ACCESSORIES

These are designed specifically to provide additional health benefits over and above those provided within the basic design of essential items. Although some are genuinely useful and helpful, others are simply gimmicks. Before buying any sort of ergonomic accessory, it is essential to consider its contribution within the overall context of the working environment. No accessory, for example, will put right a problem caused by unreasonable deadlines, keystroke-per-hour incentives, or a dull and tedious job. Accessories are really just that—an additional bonus on top of a good basic working environment.

Most accessories are specifically marketed as preventative measures of RSI, eyestrain, or emission damage. As a general rule, the simpler they are and the more modest their claims, the more likely they are to be effective. *Wrist rests* are an effective method of training users to hold their arms in a more natural alignment, avoiding the sharp wrist-arm angle so characteristic of the carpal tunnel syndrome sufferer. Such rests can be simple pads of firm, spongy material which lie along the bottom edge of the keyboard, or more sophisticated gadgets which clip on to the keyboard and can be adjusted to the individual's needs. Others come with a matching mouse rest, a smaller pad which lies on the mouse mat (or may even be built into it) and provides similar support for the mouse hand. A particularly good wrist rest uses tiny beads to create a dense pad like a beanbag. It molds around the user's wrist but provides firm support, and can be easily readjusted for different people.

With the exception of the innovative keyboards discussed above, *ergonomic keyboards* rely on subtle effects such as a slightly different degree of curvature or key travel distance from the standard model. Nonetheless, this can make a difference to those users with particularly bad typing habits. Aggressive pounders of the keyboard may benefit from a curved design which minimizes the need to stretch the fingers, and nervous "hunt and peck" typists may prefer a shorter travel distance which reduces the effort necessary to produce a contact. Any keyboard claiming to be ergonomic should include some element of wrist support, whether it be a flattened edge or a separate wrist rest included as part of the price, since wrist-related complaints are by far the most common among keyboard users. Compliance with current standards implies that keyboard design, including board shape and key spacing, has been researched and optimized.

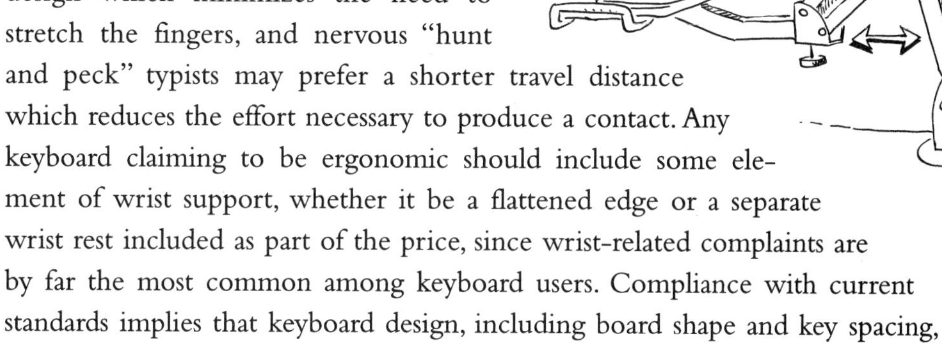

One ingenious alternative to the tilt and swivel monitor design is the *ergonomic arm*, a hinged metal arm with a tough steel spring which supports the weight of the monitor from underneath. It enables the monitor to be supported above the desk, leaving more room beneath, and increases the range of movement and precision of location of the monitor.

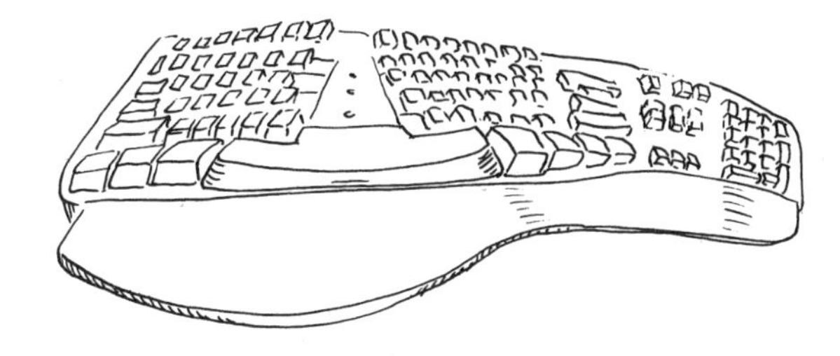

The ergonomic arm (above right) and keyboard allow for individual requirements.

Around the computer, the *document holder* represents one of the simplest but most effective ergonomic accessories. A simple panel with clip, it stands upright and enables the user to read a paper document without craning the neck or peering at a flat sheet. The benefits to the head, neck, shoulders, and eyes are immediate and significant, especially for people whose work involves substantial copy typing. If one were to buy a single ergonomic accessory for employees, the document holder would probably provide the best return on one's investment.

For the eyes and body in general, *filters* fitted over the monitor offer a range of benefits, from simple light moderation to full-scale radiation blocking. These latter filters are controversial and can be a gimmicky waste of money, often relying on people's fears for their sales. Anything which claims to reduce the level of emissions should be treated with caution, since the major source of radiation is the fly-back transformer that whips the electron beam across the screen to scan lines, and is not located near the screen but in the rear of the monitor. People sitting behind a monitor are therefore at greater risk than those actually using it, and full protection would require wrapping a shield around the entire monitor, not just the screen.

Glare filters provide a much more constructive solution to light-related problems, although even they should be considered only after the overall position of the monitor in relation to nearby windows has been optimized. The cheaper variety consists of a black nylon mesh screen, while more expensive models are made of tinted glass. Polarizing filters act just like the familiar Polaroid sunglasses, allowing only light waves vibrating in a particular plane to filter through to your eyes. Room light passes through the polarizer and strikes the screen. Reflection twists the rays one-quarter turn and the light wave is trapped, unable to pass back through the polarizer to your eyes. Anti-reflection coatings on other filters cloak the glass with multiple layers of material. If the layers are exactly the right thickness (measured in fractions of an optical wavelength), then light bouncing off the uppermost layers interferes with light bouncing off the glass substratum and destroys glare.

Some glare protectors can serve other purposes. Several companies offer mesh filters of metallic threads coated with nylon, which absorbs black light. When these are properly grounded, the conductive screens drain static electricity from the face of the monitor. The screen stays cleaner because it no longer attracts charged dust particles, and users are spared the dust that collects around the screen as it is repelled by the same charge.

PRINTERS AND PERIPHERALS

These can be among the most annoying items in terms of space and noise. Ink jet printers are noisier than laser printers, so it is important to place them as far as possible from overloaded ears. Partitions can help to muffle the din and longer cables are available to locate a printer more remotely from its users. Networks obviously enable printer sharing in offices, a sound economic move as well as helpful in keeping the noise down. Modems and CD-ROM drives are cumbersome and work as well under as on the desk, and piles of floppy disks should be stored in any of the storage boxes widely available. Although notebook personal computers might appear to represent a compact, space-saving alternative to the desktop version, they are too small for prolonged use.

SOFTWARE

Having read the sections on software in Chapter 2, you will understand that it is the most problematic buying decision for some people, many of whom tend to rely on the well-intentioned recommendations of friends or colleagues when making a choice. Choosing the right application (or suite of applications) is undeniably a complex process, but there are some ground-rules for choosing software which will support maximum productivity and minimum frustration.

The first and most important point is to involve you, the user of software, in the buying process as early and as frequently as possible. People who have choice and control in any decision will feel a strong sense of ownership and responsibility for the effects of that decision, and will work harder to make it a success.

Next, and almost as important: Be sure you *understand what you want to do* before you buy the software to do it. The range of software available today is immensely diverse, and not all of it is designed to fulfill a clear and specific need. With an unclear requirement, it is far too easy to purchase software with an unclear purpose, leaving yourself in a fog of confusion. Ascertain what tasks you perform most frequently and match these tasks to available software. Most word processors and spreadsheets now include mature and extensive abilities, so it is less critical which manufacturer you actually buy from for these applications. Software for less general tasks—stock control, accounts management, design or technical drawing, for example—is more diverse because it tends to be tailored to more specific tasks. Don't take anyone's word for it when they claim their software is the easiest to use. Read reviews and ask for demonstration or trial periods of the products you are considering.

When buying off-the-shelf applications for standard tasks, look for careful use of graphics, speech-like dialogue boxes, obvious Help, well-designed manuals, and consistent terminology. Most manufacturers offer a "suite" of applications, which do have the benefit of guaranteed consistency, a common "look and feel"—and just one person to complain to. Don't feel obligated to buy a lot of applications from one manufacturer, however. If you prefer to buy more than one package, it is in your interest to buy both, and it need not cause compatibility problems. Single or home-based users will undeniably benefit from *application suites*—they are very much cheaper than buying each member of the set separately. Although the components of a suite offer reduced functionality, in most cases the remaining functions are more than adequate for general uses.

Buyers with a tight budget should be wary about buying obscure software from very small outlets, however tempting the price, unless it is highly specialized and unlikely to be available from any other source. It is easy to turn a great idea into a nice-looking piece of code, but far more difficult to match the idea with a genuine market need, complete with all the additional functions and abilities that users now expect. You are also far more likely to turn up expensive compatibility problems with alternate products, which might not read or print files created with other packages. For their own economic good, the largest manufacturers do support each other's software. And you'll always need to be sure of reliable support for anything from an ambiguous error message to full installation. Only large manufacturers can afford to offer free, 24-hour "hotline" telephone support or engineers who arrive at your doorstep within the hour (although even the big companies are now beginning to charge for use of such support services). Finally, don't forget that software changes very rapidly and you will want a clear upgrade path well into the foreseeable future. Not all small outlets are able to sustain their investment (or interest) in a single product, which may leave you with an outdated application only six months after purchase.

Companies with a very demanding requirement, or particular way of working, may have their own software department (or prefer to employ consultants) to specify and design the software. In this case, it is the responsibility of the designers to identify and accommodate user needs, but the employer should be sure to encourage testing with "real" users as early and as frequently as possible. In any case, never underestimate the huge loss of productivity caused by badly designed, frustrating software. Too many users will not speak up because they blame themselves, so talk to designers and manufacturers about the ways they try to get around this.

For those who can afford it, formal training is a rewarding investment which gets users proficient and productive in a very short time. It is expensive, however, and the bill can hit several thousand dollars by the time you are fully trained. The solution is to be selective about your training. For applications where the concepts are well understood (such as word processors) a one-hour class in basic operation will probably be enough. For more sophisticated applications, more extensive training will be required. For employers, if you can afford to send everyone, do so, but if not, send one or two people who can then pass on the most important concepts to their colleagues. Set aside time for such exercises—if training is treated as a valuable use of one morning, the trainees will take it more seriously.

Despite claims to the contrary, there is no software with which users will be fluent the first time. Difficulties can be minimized by selecting software which includes a tutorial, either within the manual or on-line, and preferably both. The best products offer a full tutorial—or even a video—often lasting for an hour or more, plus mini-tutorials which concentrate on common problems and can be dipped into as required.

Chapter 2 outlines in more detail some of the human factors and ergonomic principles which can make the differences between software which people use and software which gathers dust on the shelf.

Healthy environmental factors

FURNITURE

This comprises the larger part of the overall work space or workstation. It is also the equipment around which our bodies will be draped for the larger part of the working day, so it is important to be comfortable. Poorly designed chairs are often implicated in back trouble and ultimately RSI, and tables which cannot accommodate the computer, its peripherals and user will lead to a cramped posture. Many manufacturers are aware of this, with the result that the term "ergonomic" has now been applied indiscriminately to a vast range of office items, many of which are little more than gimmicks. If you really want specialized ergonomic furniture, check that manufacturers' claims are endorsed. If you don't want to check the criteria individually, furniture conforming to international standard ISO9241 falls within the professionally specified range of measurements for the general population.

Chairs and desks should ideally be chosen together so that they complement one another. It is no use having the perfect chair if your desk is so low that it crushes your knees anyway. Most office desks are made to standard dimensions based on anthropometric data, arriving at a happy medium of 30 inches high. Standard office desks conform to height and depth criteria and are satisfactory for the majority of the population, but may be uncomfortable for anyone over 5'10" tall or under 5'3". The number of people in these "extreme" categories is actually quite large, with up to 50 percent of women being under 5'3". Tall people will benefit only from a higher desk—even if a chair is adjustable to their height, the effect will be back pain due to either a stooping posture or because the knees are higher than the hips. Short people require a footrest, and are now legally entitled to ask for one.

Adjustable chairs are now equally a requirement, since no set of dimensions fits everyone. The height of the seat should be adjustable between 15-21 inches, and the backrest should tilt to support the user at work and rest. Typists often prefer high-backed chairs while less intensive computer users have a preference for a more relaxed posture. The trick is to be flexible, which means having a chair that is adjustable. Swivel chairs are preferable to stationary ones, in which case the base should have five points and should include castors. It is important to test chairs to be sure that the controls are easy to operate and within reach of the seated user—and make sure you know how they work! Bear in mind that if two or more people are going to be using one work area, the equipment must be adjustable so that each can fit into his or her most comfortable working position.

WORK SPACE

This refers to the user's total working environment—chair, desk, computer, accessories, lighting, heating, and ventilation. Ultimately, it is the total combination which really influences human health and no single element can either kill or cure. For this reason, don't be fooled by companies offering expensive "ergonomic accessories" which look interesting or attractive. Applying ergonomics successfully means standing back and studying the whole picture, then applying a holistic solution. To begin with, a lot can be achieved by persuading staff to tidy up their office space. Tidily stacked boxes, clear walkways and regularly filed paperwork will solve many of the "ergonomic" problems that trouble offices. It is equally simple to reorganize desks so that telephone and computer cables cannot trip up passers-by. Most office desks now include slots or holes specifically for this purpose.

Good lighting management means avoiding excessive contrast between lit and unlit areas. An overlit office (far more common than one which is underlit) includes areas of sharp shadow and excessive glare, and you may be prone to frequent headaches. Don't position your computer so that it faces a window—the glare will be unbearable. Likewise, computers which back onto windows will force the user to sit facing the window with the sun in his or her eyes. (On the other hand, some users may find a view quite inspirational if their work requires a creative element.) For optimal positioning, have monitors positioned sideways to windows so that the light is as constant as possible. Windows should have adjustable blinds so that changing sunlight can be controlled.

Air conditioning which works is great—but if it fails, the effects can be disastrous. Employees have no control over air conditioning, a fact which, in itself, will make them more sensitive to discomfort. To reduce problems, it should be possible to open some windows or rely on alternative heat sources, such as portable heaters or radiators, if necessary.

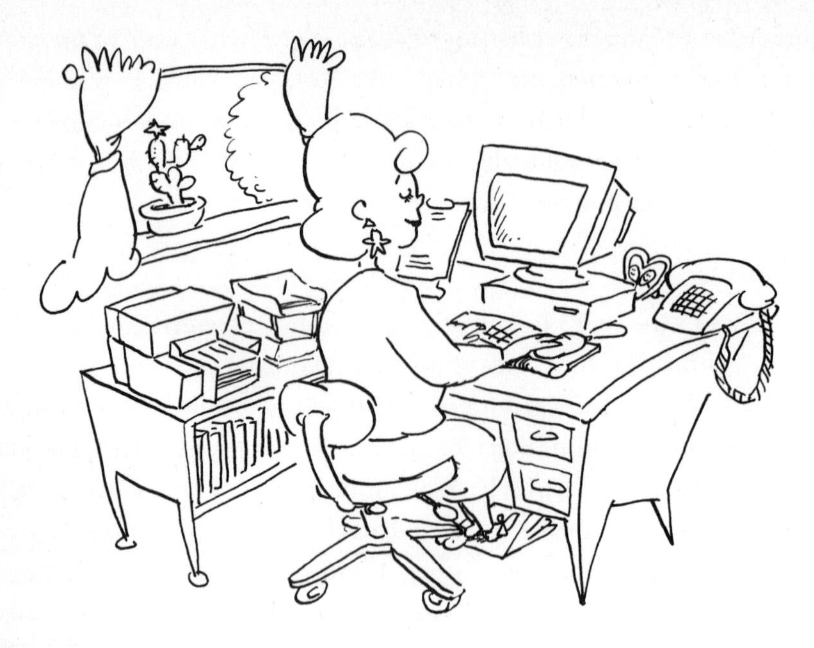

Summary of an ideal workstation layout: The desk is of a height that allows the wrists to be held naturally, and is wide enough to give room for documents and equipment; adjustable swivel chair and footrest; monitor below eye level; printer positioned to minimize noise; document holder to prevent eyestrain; papers and reference material neatly filed and easily reached.

Taking care of your environment

THE ENERGY STAR PROGRAM

More and more manufacturers are now showing concern for the overall environment, as well as the individuals who work in it. Existing initiatives are likely to become law before too long and this will almost certainly begin in the United States where the Environmental Protection Agency (EPA) launched its Energy Star Program in 1993. The EPA dates back to 1970 and is intended to control and reduce pollution, particularly with regard to air, water, solid waste, pesticides, and toxic substances. In 1992, the EPA turned its attention to the burgeoning computer industry and established a partnership between itself and as many computer and peripheral manufacturers as were interested. Those participating in the Energy Star Computers program agreed to promote the introduction of energy-efficient computer systems at no extra cost and with no loss of performance. On April 21, 1993, President Bill Clinton announced an Executive Order committing the Federal Government to purchase only equipment which complied with the specifications of the Energy Star Program. In brief, the program specifies that in order to be described as "energy efficient," a product must be able to enter a low-power state when the unit is inactive, where "low-power" means consumption of less than 30 watts for a computer, monitor, or printer producing 1 to 14 pages per minute; and less than 45 watts for color laser printers or printers with a speed greater than 15 pages per minute. Products which conform to these specifications are eligible to use the Energy Star logo in their promotional material.

The purpose of the Energy Star Program is, of course, to reduce the amount of electricity consumed by computers. This is currently estimated to absorb over five percent of the USA's annual total commercial electricity bill, rising to ten percent by the year 2000. Research by the EPA suggests that computers are being used for only a tiny proportion of the time they are actually switched on, with over a quarter of the nation's computers running overnight and on the weekend. Energy-efficient systems which "power down" when inactive stand to save the U.S. Federal Government over $40 million per year; and a further $2 billion will be lopped off the bills of American businesses. Apart from the money saved, the use of Energy Star-compliant products will reduce emissions of carbon dioxide by 20 million tons, roughly comparable to the emissions of five million cars.

In Europe, the same goals are being promoted by NUTEK, the government-owned Swedish National Board for Industrial and Technical Development. Compliance with NUTEK standards is one of several criteria which must be met in order for a monitor to qualify for "green labeling" by TCO, the powerful Swedish Confederation of Professional Employees.

POWER MANAGEMENT

The result of these drives is the emergence of *power management*, a series of measures intended to reduce electricity consumption by building automatic power down capabilities into inactive computers. There are typically two levels of power down for monitors and computers: Standby mode and sleep mode. Standby mode activates itself first after a predefined period of, say, ten minutes of continued inactivity. If a further period of inactivity, say, thirty minutes, elapses, the entire system shuts down into sleep mode. At all times, enough power is retained for the system to be reactivated by a single key press, and to maintain memory so that a user can continue working from the point at which he or she left off.

Power management was first developed for notebook computers, whose standard three-hour battery life was a frustrating limitation for travelers. Advance Power Management, developed jointly by Intel and Microsoft, comprises software which involves the operating system and applications software in the control and management of power. Variations of this technology are now being added to desktop computers to achieve compliance with Energy Star and NUTEK standards. System Management Mode is another technology which provides power management to the operating system in conjunction with low voltage (3.3 rather than 5) semiconductor chips, to eke out battery life in portables as long as possible. Finally, the development of thermostatically controlled computer cooling systems has reduced the levels of energy used for cooling, in turn reducing the air conditioning power required to balance room temperature. Flat liquid crystal displays use far less power than normal monitors, but are currently too expensive to warrant serious consideration as standard desktop equipment.

Cures: How to stop it once it has started

Despite all the precautions, some people will still develop RSI or other symptoms thought to be related to computer usage. If preventative measures don't help, or are applied too late, there are medical and paramedical treatments available which are growing in number and sophistication all the time. Don't expect miracles, however—for these injuries, cure is never as effective as prevention, and most therapists will advise holistic changes to the working environment to ensure that their individual contribution has a chance to be effective.

MEDICAL TREATMENT

The contribution of conventional medicine is relatively limited as far as the sufferers of computer-related injury, especially RSI, are concerned. Because so much of what constitutes RSI is intangible and difficult to measure, there are no formal medical treatments for the condition. In its early stages, treatment is restricted to painkillers which are not always appropriate. If corrective measures, such as micropauses or workstation redesign, are incorporated into a person's working routine, painkillers can be a suitable interim measure. They are also a good short-term solution for tension-related headache and eyestrain. Painkillers cease to be effective and can even be counterproductive if they are used for advanced cases of RSI or mild conditions which are receiving no other treatment. By dulling the pain of a chronic or serious condition, painkillers can disguise symptoms and delay the application of more appropriate treatments. They may also allow mild ailments to build up to the point where more drastic treatment is required, or even where they cannot be treated.

Medical treatment is most effective when applied to specific, localized cases of RSI, typically carpal tunnel syndrome and tenosynovitis. Sufferers of carpal tunnel syndrome demonstrate easily identifiable physical changes in the soft tissues of the wrist and hand, such as thickening of the tendon sheaths, compression of the nerves, and inflammation of the surrounding muscle. Surgery is an effective treatment for carpal tunnel syndrome: It frees tendons from the pinching of inflamed sheaths, and can ease the pressure on muscles trapped within swollen membranes. Injections of steroid-based drugs directly into the strained and swollen tendons of tenosynovitis can provide quite dramatic relief in a relatively short time, although this is not a treatment which can be used over a long period. Usually patients receiving this treatment may be offered a wrist splint to wear, which holds the wrist straight and supports them during work. Splints may be worn for days, weeks, or months, depending on the severity of the injury and the relief obtained.

MASSAGE

Massage is a broad area of therapy, and is applicable to many ailments, musculoskeletal and otherwise. It is applied directly to the soft tissues of the body—the muscles and ligaments—but has a beneficial effect over a much wider area. Techniques are generally intended to relax, strengthen, and stimulate, sometimes all at once. Massage eases tension and knotted tissue and stimulates the flow of blood and the lymphatic system. It is an important component of physical therapy and osteopathy and is used to generate a feeling of relaxed well-being.

Basic massage is usually Swedish massage, comprising a series of stroking, kneading, rolling, and squeezing techniques. Other varieties include reflexology, the massage of pressure points in the feet; and shiatsu, the Japanese technique of applying finger massage to acupuncture points of the body.

Although massage is not a specific treatment for RSI and makes no special claim to relieve or cure it, it is one of the most effective treatments for general well-being and relaxation. A trained practitioner can apply massage to relieve tension, irritability, stiffness of joints, and musculoskeletal pain, all of which can indirectly reduce the symptoms of RSI.

PHYSICAL THERAPY

Physical therapy is the treatment of physical injuries by physical means, including joint manipulation, electrotherapy, and exercise. Most physical therapists treat occupational disorders as part of their normal practice, frequently those affecting the back, upper and lower limbs, and neck and, increasingly, RSI. They are accustomed to studying and treating conditions which may not have an obvious physical cause and many of the techniques they have developed have been shown to be effective in treating RSI.

Diagnosis

Treatment from a physical therapist begins with an assessment of the condition, concentrating initially on the subjective experience of pain—the patient's choice of words to describe an injury may be as important as a physical examination in guiding the physical therapist towards a diagnosis. Some guidance is also gained from the SIN factor: The pain's Severity, its Irritability (how easily it is provoked and how long it takes to settle down), and its Nature (the likely pathology underlying it). The degree of irritability affects the intensity of the treatment, while the nature of the pain can help the therapist make important distinctions between inflammation, mechanical problems, or disease.

Using this combination of input, a physical therapist can then begin to determine whether an injury is principally neurological (involving the nerves), muscular, or articular (involving the joints); or related to posture, activity, or disease. Often it will be a combination of factors, all of which must be considered within the context of the patient's living and working environment.

Physical therapists do not regard RSI as a diagnosis in itself, but simply the description of a range of possible conditions, where precise definition and isolation is very difficult. To narrow down the possibilities, the preliminary examination will probably involve an overview of the patient's general posture; a series of simple movements which reveal ranges of joint movement; which nerves, if any, are implicated in the condition and to what extent; and a physical examination of the affected areas. If sensation is altered around the wrist or arm, the physical therapist may apply light pressure, stroking, or pinpricks to determine exactly how it is altered. He or she will check for any visible swelling or redness (indicating inflammation) and for local areas of pain. Gripping and squeezing exercises can indicate the level of muscle strength, which may in turn provide a clue to the effectiveness of the nerve supply to that area.

Treatment

The treatment of diffuse RSI can vary widely, depending on the musculoskeletal and neurological systems involved, the extent of injury, the context in which pain is felt and the appearance of any physical indications of injury. Typical treatments used to relieve the symptoms of RSI include:

Joint mobilization and manipulation. Often this technique will be applied to joints in the neck and upper trunk, which are effectively a channel for many of the body's major nerve networks. The intention is to correct the alignment of the head and neck in relation to the rest of the body; to release nerves which may be compressed or pinched (transmitting pain down to the arm and hand); and to relax and realign the muscles of the neck and shoulder which will in turn encourage a more natural posture of the wrist and arm. Where appropriate, joint mobilization may be applied to the shoulder, elbow, and wrist.

Nerve mobilization. If the physical therapist believes the underlying problem to be adverse mechanical tension in the nervous system, the treatment can include some element of mobilization of the appropriate nerves. Where it is thought that the nerve is rubbing on or being pulled against another tissue by faulty action of that tissue, the affected tissue (bone, muscle, or tendon) will also be treated to reduce the chance of recurrence of nerve-related problems.

Pain relievers. These are not the drug-based treatments of mainstream medicine but other techniques and treatments designed to relieve pain. Straightforward massage may be used to induce a greater level of overall relaxation and feeling of well-being, or heat-based therapies can be used for the same effect. Some physical therapists may use acupuncture to relax muscles, increase circulation, and reduce pain levels.

Electrotherapy. Ultrasound and laser and inferential treatments can be applied to stimulate or sedate the peripheral nervous system, increase local blood circulation to an affected area and stimulate the body's healing processes.

Drug treatment. Not generally the province of physical therapists, drug treatments take the form of oral anti-inflammatory medication or localized cortisone injections to a specific area. These drugs can be effective in the short term, and are similar to those described as part of medical treatment.

Work visits. Physical therapists will often arrange to visit the patient's workplace to analyze his or her work tasks and assess their likely contribution to the symptoms. They may suggest changes in the task, the workstation, or the tools to minimize irritation to a current injury, or to prevent future ones.

OSTEOPATHY

Osteopathy focuses closely on the body's musculoskeletal system and is most often associated with the treatment of back pain and spinal injuries. Some osteopaths extend their areas of expertise and treatment into other complaints of the musculoskeletal system, including respiratory, gastrointestinal, and cardiovascular disturbance while others handle occupational health disorders such as RSI. Like physical therapists, osteopaths begin their diagnosis with a detailed interview covering the patient's medical history; the nature and characteristics of the complaint; and a physical examination. The examination includes a number of standard clinical procedures which will enable the osteopath to determine how appropriate osteopathic treatment is and how likely the patient is to benefit.

Diagnosis

Wherever the location of musculoskeletal pain, an osteopath will use palpation and manipulative techniques to explore levels of overall muscle tension and the quality of spinal function in detail, since osteopaths tend to hold the view that musculoskeletal pain in any area of the body may be indirectly related to spinal function. For a localized injury, fingertip exploration can reveal specific areas and types of tension, muscle spasm and pain. The interview will often involve a thorough discussion of the patient's life habits, to build up a comprehensive picture of the factors which may contribute to the injury. Because of their expertise in the treatment of back pain, osteopaths are not strangers to conditions which show no quantifiable symptoms and cannot readily be explained. This makes them sensitive therapists for the RSI sufferer and, like physical therapists, they are adept at drawing together the diverse contributory factors which underlie RSI.

If the osteopath decides that a patient is suffering from diffuse RSI and will benefit from osteopathic treatment, he or she will try to understand more about the patient's working life and habits. This may, in turn, reveal small—or even obvious—changes that could be made at once to provide relief.

Treatment

Again depending on the nature, severity, and location of a computer-related injury, osteopathic treatment can vary widely. General treatments may be direct or indirect, and osteopaths seek to treat the whole person rather than a specific part.

Direct treatment. This approach covers all treatments which are applied directly to the injury. Soft tissue manipulation is a massaging and relaxation of the muscles with special focus on localized areas of tension. A more widespread injury may require articulatory techniques, whereby the osteopath moves the patient's affected joints through a series of stretching exercises. For some specific conditions, high velocity thrust techniques can be applied—sudden, firm movements of the spine which may cause a snapping noise, although this is rarely appropriate for computer-related injury.

Indirect treatment. Less widely used, these techniques involve the application of passive force to areas of injury until a release of movement is obtained. They may also involve the massage of areas, particularly the head, neck, and spine, with a view to freeing movement in other areas such as limbs.

Specific treatments of RSI. Much of what osteopaths have to offer RSI sufferers overlaps substantially with the treatment of the physical therapist. Joint and tissue mobilization is a common treatment, although in very general terms osteopaths concentrate more on the neck and spine and the trigger points of major muscles. One of the most beneficial aspects of osteopathy is that it actively attempts to provide treatments which the patient can perform at home. This provides the element of control which is known to be important to an effective cure and means that it can be applied when required. "Cupping" can also be a simple and effective treatment, whereby a small plastic cup is placed over a tender or spasmodic muscle. This creates a vacuum, and when the cup is lifted, helps lift the tissues in the area and free blood flow.

Treatments which can be applied at home are not exclusive to osteopaths; they and other therapists may prescribe less common treatments found to be effective in individual cases. *Thalassotherapy*, for example, is the treatment of an injury with cold and hot sea water and can easily be applied at home. The injured area (usually the lower arm, wrist, and hand) is plunged into very cold and then very hot water repeatedly for a ten-minute period, which increases the blood flow to that area and relaxes the muscle.

POSTURAL TRAINING

Good therapists acknowledge that their specialized contribution to the treatment of RSI can have only a short-term effect at best if the overall health and mental attitude of the patient is not basically sound. One of the most holistic therapies of benefit to RSI sufferers is postural training, an approach to the human organism as a whole entity, which does not address a specific complaint but is nevertheless remarkably helpful to a range of conditions related to the musculoskeletal system.

The Alexander Technique

One of the best known and most effective postural training techniques is the Alexander technique, named after its founder, F. M. Alexander. Alexander was an actor in the latter part of the nineteenth century whose promising career was threatened by vocal troubles with no apparent medical cause. He began to observe himself in the mirror during speaking and noticed he had a tendency to stiffen his neck and pull his head back and down, depressing his vocal cords and shortening his spine. By consciously training himself to hold his head in correct alignment with his neck and torso, he overcame the problem. He passed his discovery on to other actors who reported other, unforeseen health benefits they had achieved, and by the turn of the century Alexander had given up acting in favor of the development and teaching of his new postural training technique.

Alexander believed that many cases of "dis-ease" were attributable to the misuse of the body rather than any fault of the body itself. He made a careful study of human physiology to support this idea, and many subsequent researchers have confirmed some of his theories. For example, it has now been shown that different muscle types are perfectly adapted to different functions—some "fast" muscles are adapted to short bursts of high energy, producing peak levels of exertion but tiring easily. "Slow" muscle cannot provide these bursts, but is better adapted to supporting the body in one position for many hours at a time. Many postural problems are related to the use of fast muscle for long-term, "slow" supporting functions, which is fatiguing and reduces tone and efficiency in slow muscles. Similarly, many people sit in a way which places a far greater load on the ligaments than the muscles themselves, straining and damaging connective tissues.

The basic concept underlying the Alexander technique is that the human body is perfectly adapted to the upright position, although few of us actually use our bodies correctly. When we do, the effect is perfect balance and poise with a minimum degree of tension. Lessons in the Alexander technique attempt to reveal, through touch and explanation, what a person's postural problems are and how they are interfering with the head-neck-torso relationship in rest and activity. A large part of the training concerns attitude—students are encouraged to become more aware of their own bodily posture and to consciously adopt new habits of bearing and coordination. Many students report sensations of the body lengthening and lightening even after one lesson, with many gross movements become effortless. The technique is rarely applied to very specific postural defects, since Alexander saw his work as a holistic treatment for the whole organism. Specific problems, he believed, required specific attention to the conditions which gave rise to them. In addition, he acknowledged the importance of practice and the conscious effort his technique required, and regarded it as a re-education in movement which had to be learned. Although the benefits are apparent after only one lesson, they will be short-lived if the pupil does not continue to learn and apply him or herself afterwards to the conscious development of the Alexander technique.

For this reason, the Alexander technique cannot be regarded as a "cure" for RSI, or indeed any other musculoskeletal complaint. It is a holistic approach to movement and bearing which can prevent and indirectly relieve many complaints, traditionally back and neck-related, which have arisen over the years. For RSI sufferers, an understanding of the technique may improve their seated and working postures to the extent that neck and upper limb pain cease to be problems, gradually eliminating the more specific effects of RSI. It should also be noted that the Alexander technique can be of little benefit to conditions such as carpal tunnel syndrome or tenosynovitis, where there are specific pathological changes to body tissues. It is likely to be of the greatest benefit to patients suffering from diffuse RSI across the upper limb, neck, and shoulders, where specific treatments seem inappropriate and there are no pathological changes which can be addressed.

Which therapy is the most effective treatment for RSI?

There is no easy answer. Repetitive strain injury has a wide range of complex causes and any single sufferer will be the victim of an infinite variety of subtle factors and influences. Postural training will provide a holistic preventative treatment, but it will only work if other, broader working conditions are attended to as well. Physical therapy and osteopathy can offer more specific treatments for diagnosed conditions, but it is impossible to tell in advance which will be the most appropriate. Some general practioners will have the knowledge and experience to refer patients to a more appropriate practitioner while others will be unfamiliar with RSI and may only prescribe painkillers, thus masking the problem. The solution is a combination of initiative and trial and error. If your general practioner seems uncertain about treatment for RSI, ask for a referral to a physical therapist or osteopath. Neither of these professionals should begin treatment without gaining a clear understanding of your working conditions and practices; if they do, it is probably worth getting a second opinion.

Depending on the physical mechanisms implicated in your condition, different therapists will offer more or less effective treatments. Any professional worth his or her salt will recognize a condition which requires the knowledge of an alternative practitioner, and will refer you accordingly. Summon up the courage to try a different treatment if you don't feel the one you are receiving is adequate, but bear in mind the effect of psychological factors on your condition. It may be that no physical treatment is enough to correct the problems of a menial and soul-destroying job.

Eye care

Like the rest of the body, the eyes are composed of tissues, fibers, and muscles which get tired when they are used for intensive work over a long period of time. Many people are alarmed to find that their eyes are tired at the end of a day in front of the computer, but this is simply the natural result of extended, intensive visual work in a demanding environment. Visual fatigue is just as uncomfortable as muscular fatigue can be, perhaps more so since tired eyes become dry, red, and sore.

The first step towards reducing eyestrain is to have your eyes tested by an ophthalmologist. This will identify any preexisting visual problems which may be exacerbated by staring at a monitor and ensure the provision of any corrective appliances immediately. Employers are now obliged to pay for their employees to take an eye test, and will pay for any appliance required as a result of monitor usage. See Chapter 8 for more details on your rights in this area. Assuming your eyes are fine (or that existing defects have been corrected), the next step is to optimize the working environment, especially lighting and glare.

The best lighting compromise is diffuse overhead lighting supplemented by focused spotlights for document reading. Natural light is still easiest on the eye, but use blinds to control sun rays and align the monitor at right angles to windows where possible, to minimize changes to the level of light. The virtues of glare screens are discussed in the section on ergonomic accessories (p. 120).

However well-lit it is, a poor quality monitor will definitely aggravate eyestrain and it may be worth demanding or investing in a better one if you are a regular user. Visually beneficial replacements have a flatter screen which is less likely to pick up extraneous light sources and is therefore less prone to glare.

Another simple step to combat eye fatigue is to clear away dust on a regular basis. Monitor screens naturally attract dust because the high voltage used by their electron beams builds up a static charge on the face of the tube. If you don't have a reduced electrostatic charge monitor, use a damp rag and a squirt of anti-static spray to wipe dust gently off the screen. Be careful not to get the screen really wet, as any liquid that runs down its face can drip inside and damage the monitor's circuitry.

Eyes will become more fatigued if you have to look up at the monitor, since your eyes are wider open and feel dryer more quickly. As previously stated, the optimum height for the monitor is such that the top of the screen is at eye level and the eyes gaze down at an angle of around 15 degrees. It also helps to have some kind of stand or holder for reference material during typing. To minimize eye fatigue, keep whatever you are typing from at the same distance from your eyes as the monitor screen so that you don't have to shift focus every time you check your notes. Less shifting of focus is believed to minimize fatigue. Periodically, however, you should take a break and shift your focus. Think of it as a visual micropause; look around the office or out of the window, or gaze at a distant horizon—anything to change focus and relax your eyes. As with arms and wrists, the way to minimize eyestrain, fatigue, and irritation is to moderate visual work. Don't shift your focus dozens of times a minute, and don't lock your eyes at a consistent distance for hours on end.

Some optometrists recommend "palming" as a therapeutic technique for eyes. Rub the hands together to generate some warmth, then place cupped hands over your eyes, palms inwards. Use the heel of the hand and fleshy pad at the base of the fingers to massage the cheek bone and brow bone in small, gentle, circular movements, keeping the eyes open if possible. Do this for a minute or so. Palming relieves tension around the eye area and gives the eyes a rest by preventing them from focusing for the duration of the treatment. It is simple to learn and can be applied whenever it is required.

Learning to cope with stress at work

THE WEAK LINK

The factor which underpins so many of the computer-related health problems discussed in this book is stress. It is not restricted to computer users either: Many doctors believe that stress plays a vital part in the development of all illnesses, both physical and mental. The exact mechanisms are not known but, broadly speaking, researchers believe that a high level of stress—or even a low level maintained over a long period—disturbs normal body functioning and makes us vulnerable to all sorts of health problems. Exactly what sort of problem develops depends very much on the individual, making it that much more difficult to determine whether stress is a factor. Many healthy people suffer from an increase in headaches, sore throats, or digestive difficulties. Other people, perhaps with a history of eczema or blood pressure, may find their medical problems exacerbated during times of stress; still others whose stress has an emotional element (perhaps arguments at home or work), may experience depression or irrational outbursts of anger. In any case, it is becoming more and more apparent to researchers that a strong correlation between mind and body does exist.

The common factor is that it is the "weak link" in a person that is most likely to break in times of stress. Hence, computer users whose "weak link" is likely to be cramped and strained muscles in the upper limbs are more liable to develop RSI. People who stare at the screen in an incorrect angle or for extended periods are more prone to eyestrain and headaches; and so on.

It is certainly possible that an individual under no particular stress will develop a computer-related injury, but this is unlikely to be serious or prolonged. Truly debilitating RSI rarely occurs in a situation where the sufferer is happy and fulfilled at work. Likewise, where feelings of satisfaction and achievement are low, many people will report symptoms.

Stress and all that it implies—unhappiness, a lack of control, poor adaptation to an environment or way of doing things, failures, and disappointments—is a powerful predictor of illness. It therefore makes sense to understand and-preempt stress before it leads to the breaking of the weak link.

Tactics for tackling stress at work

This section deals with the everyday hassle that affects all of us much of the time. It does not deal with the comparatively rare events that can be shattering, such as the death of a loved one, break-up of a relationship, or loss of a job. These events can rarely be prepared for and there are no rules about coping: They need to be dealt with sensitively and appropriately, depending on the individual and the circumstances.

EVALUATING SITUATIONS MORE POSITIVELY

Whether or not people feel under stress may depend largely on how they perceive their situation. Many actually do find it helps to regard "problems" as "challenges" or "opportunities." Learning to evaluate potentially stressful situations in a more positive light can make them less stressful—it is often simply a case of thinking about things in a different way. For example, a monotonous data entry job can undoubtedly be a source of stress, although the degree of stress will vary according to the way employees perceive it. The person who regards such a job as an insult to his or her intelligence, a waste of time, or a futile exercise will certainly be unhappier than the employee who sees it as a break from domesticity, a source of income, or a chance to plan ways of achieving more demanding employment.

This may sound like nothing more than optimism, but there are ways of learning to develop new, more positive evaluations of potentially stressful or frightening situations: For every fear there is a corresponding opportunity. A positive outlook is more rational and calming than a negative one, turning a terrifying ordeal into quite a career opportunity. Nothing about the situation has changed, but by forcing oneself to articulate the potential for success behind the fear, it becomes decidedly less formidable. At the very least, you should ask yourself: *Even if everything I can imagine goes wrong, shall I still be worrying about it in one, three, or five year's time?* If the answer is no, it is really not that big a problem. Tackle stress by bringing it into your consciousness; take time to really think about troublesome issues and make decisions about dealing with them. They are rarely as bad as they seem.

Gaining Competency and Confidence

It would be more difficult to find a positive side to the situation if one was unable to derive any meaning from the work demanded. This might be the fault of the person in charge, but it might be that an employee simply lacks the competence, training, or experience to deal with what is expected of her. Feeling that one is not up to the task is a source of great stress and can undermine self-confidence drastically.

It is obviously not sensible to apply for a job for which you have no appropriate qualifications. More typically, an employer might ask employees (deliberately or unintentionally) to perform tasks which they are simply not capable of doing. Computer operators with no keyboard training will find a data entry task far more difficult than their keyboard-trained colleagues; similarly, even confident new graduates are unlikely to manage a team of executives with the skill of a senior manager. It is important to be aware of one's capabilities and limitations and negotiate working responsibilities accordingly. If the job demands a new skill, training should be provided or allowance made for inexperience. Feeling competent to meet one's responsibilities reduces stress and promotes self-confidence.

Gaining Control and Diminishing Helplessness

Early psychological experiments on stress showed that animals who believe they cannot escape an electric shock will soon cease to try. Eventually, they will continue passively to receive shocks, even when an escape route is made available to them. In other words, they learn to be helpless in the face of unpleasant, stressful events over which they have no control. People can respond in the same way over a period of time—if they believe they have no control whatsoever over the stressful things happening to them, they will eventually stop trying to resist. Feelings of helplessness or powerlessness will crush initiative and prevent employees from developing feelings of commitment to or involvement in their work, damaging overall levels of quality and productivity.

Gaining control is not about seizing power, it is more about increasing the cooperation between employers and employees to make people feel more involved in decisions and choice. A supervisor might set weekly targets instead of hourly ones, leaving employees to decide their own interim targets and allocate their own break periods. More staff members might be invited to attend meetings where strategic decisions are made, or employees might be asked to contribute suggestions for improvement to their working conditions at regular intervals. Obviously, employees cannot gain more control over their work without the cooperation of employers and supervisors, and this subject is discussed in more detail in the section on job design (p. 147).

GIVING AND RECEIVING SUPPORT

A degree of social support in the working environment is one of the best ways to mitigate stress. People with supportive family and friends are far less likely to suffer from illness than those who have no social support, and the ability to talk about worrisome issues to an understanding confidante is key to this. Support enables a person to place stressful events in a broader context and perceive them as less dominant, whereas the more isolated worker may dwell on problems and focus unnecessary anxiety on a relatively trivial event.

If social support is not available, it may be necessary to provide more formal support structures at work. Some organizations use a "mentoring scheme," whereby more senior staff adopt the semi-formal role of mentor to more junior staff. A mentor is not necessarily the junior's immediate superior and may fulfill an unrelated job function, but there is normally some element of common ground. The mentor acts as the junior's advisor, supporter, and teacher, spending time talking through work experiences and problems and recommending possible solutions. In some cases, the mentor may be only a year or two older than the junior, and is thus able to offer insights from more recent personal experience.

Larger organizations may employ part- or full-time counselors to provide a confidential counseling service to employees. This rarely has a psychological or medical bias and is more likely to offer career or professional advice as the primary service. Counseling on personal and emotional matters is generally available as part of the service, however.

LEARNING TO RELAX

Stress causes physical and mental tension, and by relieving these tensions it is possible to reduce stress. Relaxation techniques have been thoroughly studied over recent years, with many researchers reporting significant benefits as a result. Practiced regularly, relaxation techniques appear to have a cumulative beneficial effect. Common relaxation techniques include meditation, relaxation tapes, hypnosis, biofeedback, and cognitive coping strategies.

Meditation is perhaps the simplest relaxation technique. At its most basic, it involves moving to a calm place, sitting quietly, perhaps with closed eyes, breathing deeply, and clearing the mind. Over just five minutes it is possible to lower the blood pressure, dissipate feelings of frustration and anger, and achieve greater muscle relaxation. More formal meditation techniques are sometimes taught and often draw on eastern religious practices or exercises such as yoga. Such techniques may teach ways of clearing the mind, methods of concentration, focus, and problem resolution. Chanting may be part of the technique, or gentle movements. Meditation offers different experiences depending on the level at which it is practiced and, clearly, an hour's meditation using a taught technique will confer greater benefit than a five-minute deep breathing exercise. That said, five-minute slots are more likely to occur during the working day than one-hour periods and, practiced regularly, will have a cumulative beneficial effect.

Relaxation tapes contain soothing music, relaxing imagery, and sometimes subliminal messages to calm the listener. Less demanding than meditation, they can be played at leisure and require only that you listen and learn to relax. Obviously they cannot be used in an office, but make a delightful accompaniment to a quiet evening alone or a hot bath. Tapes containing subliminal messages should always state the contents of the message on the cover.

The medical and psychological benefits of *hypnosis* are well-documented and have been applied to a wide range of conditions. The principle by which hypnosis operates is not that of the trance, as many popular portrayals suggest, but of deep relaxation. Using hypnotic techniques, a trained hypnotist (more commonly called a hypnotherapist nowadays) can induce in patients a feeling of intense well-being and relaxation. In this state, it is possible to reach resources in the mind which are normally blocked or inhibited and bring them into play in an individual's everyday life. Dieting, giving up smoking, and conquering minor psychosomatic illnesses are common applications of hypnotherapy. Hypnosis will not reduce stress directly, but can enable a patient to learn techniques of relaxation gradually, reproducing them more readily at will.

Biofeedback is a relatively complex (and now rarely used) technique which, once learned, can prove beneficial. As the name suggests, it involves the patient receiving direct input about the state of his or her mind and body, displayed graphically and electronically. Using electrodes, sphygnamometers and other physiological measurement techniques, it is possible to record the progress of heart rate, blood pressure, breathing rate, sweating, and skin sensitivity as an individual experiences different levels of stress. By observing that heart rate increases as stress levels rise, for example, it becomes easier for a person to concentrate on slowing his or her heart rate, keeping breathing even and hence minimizing the experience of stress. At first, it is difficult to control these responses, but with time and practice—and feedback—it is possible to develop remarkable control of these "semi-automatic" processes.

For those with little time to relax physically, stress can be alleviated by developing *cognitive coping strategies*. This involves altering one's thinking and attitudes to evaluate situations more positively, as discussed above. Some therapists can teach techniques for developing such strategies, by concentrating on recent examples of stress in an individual's life. Learning cognitive coping strategies concentrates on focusing on specific thoughts as they occur in a stressful situation, examining them, and replacing them with more rational, positive statements. In time, it becomes easier to approach stress in a more positive frame of mind.

For employers: Redesigning the workplace to increase involvement, control, productivity, and health

It is obviously in everyone's interest to pursue practices which reduce stress, keep everyone happy, and maintain the interest, involvement, and health of everyone concerned. Although treatments are available for RSI, visual discomfort, and similar complaints, prevention is generally preferable. At one level, this can be achieved by designing workstations to take account of ergonomics, usability, and environmental comfort; at another level, the individual can contribute by taking preventative steps to reduce the risk of and vulnerability to computer-related health problems. At the broadest possible level, this can be achieved by reducing the chances of employees falling prey to feelings of boredom, apathy, alienation, detachment, and a lack of control over any part of the job. As previous chapters have shown, these feelings commonly occur in sufferers of RSI, electrical hypersensitivity, skin rash, and a wide range of minor complaints—headaches, blurred vision, and so forth. While not a direct cause, they are undoubtedly a contributory factor to health problems, and any steps which can be taken to address these issues are certain to reduce the incidence of computer-related health problems. Quite possibly, maintaining employees' interest, involvement, and satisfaction will have a positive impact on every aspect of their lives. The concept of *job design* attempts to address these questions. Not originally intended to deal with any specific health problem, it nevertheless operates at a sufficiently broad level to counter many elements of occupational disorder.

The notion of designing jobs around human capabilities, rather than vice versa, dates back to the 1920s. At that time, many management theorists were of the opinion that workers were by nature lazy and untrustworthy and needed discipline and management at all times. From this point of view, control was clearly something only managers should be allowed to handle. To this end, the concept of "scientific management" emerged, a theory which prescribed systematic work procedures, greatly simplified and highly specified. Each process in a work flow was broken down into its smallest elements—for example, a manufacturing process would be broken down into the details of component sorting, assembling, checking, testing, and packing. Each worker would be assigned an exact number of these elements with no deviation from the assigned tasks. The entire process was tightly controlled by supervisors. Scientific management was designed both to prevent exploitation of workers by the management, and deceit and laziness by workers. Unlike more modern theories, however, it reduced the human role to that of mindless robots who take no part in decision-making and have no conception of what the end-products of their labors might be.

In the 1950s and '60s, further research into occupational health began to cast off the early influence of scientific management. Instead, a series of studies by the Tavistock Institute began to show more clearly that such mindless and repetitive jobs are dehumanizing and reduce productivity. There followed a range of motivational theories, elements of which are still influential today, and ultimately the notion of work as a complex *sociotechnical system*. This term encapsulated the idea of employment as more than simply a means of earning money. Researchers began to realize that jobs also provide individuals with a sense of identity, a structure to their day, a means of social contact, and a focus for aspiration and ambitions. Where these needs were adequately met, employees tended to work harder and more productively, demonstrated enthusiasm for and commitment to their work, and described their jobs as a source of personal satisfaction and self-esteem. On the basis of this evidence, many employers have begun to look more carefully at the components of employees' jobs, with a view to maximizing both employee satisfaction and productivity.

Job design in today's workplace means enlarging and enriching the task variety, responsibilities, and social interactions of employees. This does not mean turning everyone into a manager of sorts—indeed, many people actively wish to avoid excessive responsibility—but seeks instead to provide an appropriate level of stimulation for different groups of workers. For the data entry clerk, whose work may involve little more than the monotonous typing of meaningless data, job redesign might involve less typing and more filing (task variety); the typing of wider and more meaningful range of data types (task enlargement); or the opportunity to choose which of a number of possible tasks will be worked on for a given period (greater autonomy).

The feeling of being valued and of making a worthwhile commitment is enhanced by evidence of employers' investment in individuals. This need not mean higher salaries; high pay-back investments include access to training, regular and constructive performance evaluations, greater employee involvement in strategic or decision-making meetings, support of small, autonomous work groups and regular, formal feedback sessions discussing individual and group contributions to the whole operation.

CHANGE-MANAGEMENT AND JOB DESIGN FOR COMPUTER USERS

The notion of job design is clearly beneficial to many types of work at many levels, irrespective of the role that computers play. In fact, the original concept of job design saw new technology as a direct attack on the prized job characteristics of satisfaction, commitment, and involvement. Computers represent a unique problem to the employer anxious to maximize employee satisfaction, since they are so often introduced to reduce or even eliminate human contribution. Automation, whether as part of the manufacturing process in a factory or the data management system of a large corporation, all too often reduces the need for people to think, plan, design, or manage.

Clearly, the argument in favor of computers is that automation takes over the drudgery and leaves the creative work to the people. In reality, however, automation often takes over from people altogether, leaving them with nothing. It is obviously unrealistic to expect competing corporations to sacrifice vital technological advances in favor of employee happiness, but it is equally desirable that technology be introduced in a way which limits the extent to which jobs are "deskilled" and continues to make the most of human input. The process of deskilling is often gradual rather than sudden, removing power and involvement from employees and placing it more firmly in the control of senior management levels. The full nature and implications of this process are beyond the scope of the present discussion, but it seems likely that whatever relief from drudgery computers provide, they will also reduce opportunities for creative and stimulating employment at many levels. In the long term, the solution will probably require profound changes in our expectations of work and leisure, but in the short term, the introduction of new technology to the workplace demands sensitive management of change.

Good change-management is neither easy nor cheap. Far too often, automation is left to a handful of technical "experts" whose very expertise precludes a real understanding of the human issues involved. Lacking technical understanding, non-computer-literate managers often fear the technology themselves and do not contribute the planning necessary to reduce employee resistance. Leaving it to the last minute is asking for trouble, however—change-management should start when new technology is only in the system design stage, and when the initial scoping and planning are still underway. Resistance comes, unsurprisingly, from people who fear that new technology will cost them their jobs or make them look incompetent. As with other major changes, these fears can be preempted by allowing employees to participate and "buy in" to company decisions at an early stage. People at the lower echelons of an organization will otherwise feel they are being dictated to and will become accordingly resentful. To avoid rejection (and, consequently, low morale, which can be devastating to productivity), it is important for someone to "sell" new ideas and concepts to them. This may be an individual within the organization but it is equally likely that companies will need to hire change-management experts specifically to control this process. Essential skills are the ability to persuade, sell, and motivate, coupled with the technological skills to explain what they are trying to implement.

All the components of change-management have to start well before the new system is finally delivered. Trial runs of proposed systems give users a feel for what the new system will be like to use, and what it will do for them—as well as providing an opportunity to change it to meet more of their needs, more easily. Continuous support and training encourage exploration and acceptance, and may provide users with an opportunity to identify additions or alternatives to their existing roles for themselves as the system becomes a part of their working environment. Widespread automation is always threatening, but where employees are able to see it coming, influence its progress and help redefine their own contribution to the organization, they are far less likely to reject it. In this case, job redesign needs to ensure that employees retain control over when and how tasks are done; that they still have a significant component of intellectual effort in their jobs and that the availability and quality of social and professional relationships is maintained.

Job design and change-management cannot conceal the fact that the introduction of computers throughout an entire organization may render whole strata of jobs obsolete. Quite how this is resolved depends very much on the size, business, culture, and fortunes of the organization concerned, although even here there are steps which can be taken to reduce human costs. Computing and communications technology can be used to allow more employees to work more flexible hours or at different locations (including home), reducing space and rental overheads. Access to training can spread the expertise across a larger number of people, limiting the threatening concentration of power in the hands of a few specialists and increasing the contribution of others.

Summary

By far the best treatment for computer-related injury is prevention. It is more effective, lasts longer, and costs less, and the earlier it is implemented the more effective it will be. Prevention covers a range of options, from small details such as the purchase of a document holder or swivel chair, to far broader approaches which tackle the relationship of an entire job to an individual's emotional and physical health.

Prevention begins with an understanding of the computer-user in relation to his or her entire working environment. The increasing availability of ergonomically designed computing equipment, furniture, and accessories has made it easier for employers to design a safe and comfortable work place, and new legislation is now in place to ensure that employee health remains a priority issue. It is by no means the entire story, however. Despite the advantages of ergonomic design, the benefits will be limited if they are accompanied by attention to the "fit" between employee and occupation. The way in which information technology is planned and introduced to an organization can be crucial in determining employee attitudes towards computers—whether they are perceived as a threat or as a useful additional tool. The more positively employees regard computers, the more likely it is that they will attempt to learn, understand, and integrate the computer into their working routines. Positive attitudes can be encouraged by involving employees, wherever possible, in the planning and choosing of equipment early on in the process.

Users can help themselves to ward off computer-related complaints by acquiring "preventative habits"—taking short, regular breaks, maintaining an awareness of body posture, and keeping desk and office space tidy. Careful reviews of an entire office, as well as the working areas of individuals, can indicate what (if any) specific improvements can be made to the working environment to optimize the use of available equipment, and highlight areas where modifications may be required. Since the most insidious factor underlying computer-related injury (and many other health complaints) is stress, it makes sense to address this problem directly through employer-employee cooperation. It is important to remove or reduce sources of stress while simultaneously encouraging employees to develop methods of tackling potentially stressful situation before they arise. These are many and varied, but a mixture of formal and informal anti-stress measures routinely applied can enable everyone to cope better.

If old habits have already led to health problems, there are cures available. Like preventative treatments, these range from the highly specific to the very general, depending on the nature of the complaint. Medical treatment is limited but a range of paramedical therapies—physical therapy, osteopathy, and massage, for example—have proved tremendously effective in treating work-related disorders of the upper limbs, neck, and back. Invariably, these treatments are more effective and longer lived when combined with a review and overhaul of personal working habits and the immediate working environment.

The complexity and variety of factors leading to computer-related health disorders is matched by a diversity of preventative treatments and cures. No single factor is more important than any other in causing health problems and no single treatment will prevent or cure it more effectively than any other. Computer-related health complaints can only be understood, diagnosed, and treated in a very broad context, and understanding this is the first step towards a healthier working life.

CHAPTER 7

Children's Health and Computing

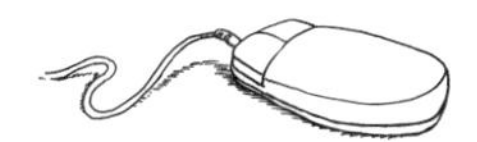

WHILE SOME ADULTS ARE NERVOUS about computers and reluctant to use them, some children cannot be torn away from them. As computers appear more and more frequently in the home, more and younger children have access to them. The computer is become something that families share—less of a tool than a recreational facility—and manufacturers are beginning to move in on this new family market for computer hardware, software, and accessories. Interacting with a computer is not always a comfortable or pleasant task, but this does not appear to be the case when a ten-year-old is seated in front of one. Children's relationships with computers can be baffling and sometimes of concern to teachers and parents, but is this just the result of poor understanding—or is it justified?

At the time of writing, people of a certain age (say, thirty-something) are unlikely to have encountered computers much before the age of twenty unless they possess an exceptional enthusiasm. Older people will not have met them until their careers were well-established, and some people simply cannot see a place for computers in the workplace at all. The response of an adult to his or her first computer depends very much on this prior experience—the more that has been achieved without computers, the less necessary (and hence the more threatening) they will appear to be.

For children, computers are far less extraordinary. Many children today are growing up with them—either their older siblings or parents use them regularly, or their friends play games on them. Computers, therefore, begin to assume the normality of a television or family car, something well-understood, whose role and purpose in everyday life is known and taken for grated. The application of computers to the business world in later life will not be a surprise but will be expected, and many of the fears and adaptations experienced by the current working population simply will not apply. Apple, the manufacturer of exceptionally friendly Apple computers, has video evidence of children as young as two years old displaying a clear understanding and skilled use of a mouse to open a drawing application and create some colorful scribbles. Amazed parents testify to the ability of their eight-year-olds to grasp the basics of computer operation and write simple programs, and many students now rely on computers to produce coursework. Educational computer software is flourishing alongside home-based applications for calculating what you have got in your bank account—and how much you owe to the tax man.

Office automation is not the burning interest of many children however, for whom entire corporations are now designing and developing software. The explosion of video games for both the television and the computer is nothing short of phenomenal and the technology now exists to convert the humble television into a vividly illustrated other world in which children can disappear for hours. Consoles, portable game units, and the games themselves have become expensive and highly coveted objects, influencing children's social and emotional life. For increasing numbers of children, "gaming" is what computing is really about.

The seductive world of video games

The appeal of video games software is simply incomprehensible to many adults, and relies greatly on the level of cognitive, emotional, and social development of many of its target market. Video games are designed to appeal to children between the ages of eight and sixteen (although there is plenty of variation of either side, as many exasperated wives will explain), and takes into accounts their needs and interests. Children in this age group are undergoing dramatic physiological and psychological changes. At the younger end, they are beginning to assert their identity as separate from their parents, develop more stable friendships and clearer gender roles, and experience the responsibility of homework. Older children are dealing with the turbulence of adolescence, self-consciousness, tentative relationships with the opposite sex, and conflict with parental wishes; while older adolescents are struggling with personal identity, self-knowledge, sexual encounters, and career issues. This period also sees the development of personal morality—an understanding of what is right and wrong—and the search for a role model from whom to derive acceptable behavior patterns.

The common theme is conflict, change, and growth, when children are particularly vulnerable to external influences on their perceptions of what is acceptable. They may feel powerless and subject to the wishes of authority figures for no clear reason; they may be wrestling with loneliness, boredom, and confusion, or lack the resources to pursue conventional entertainment. As customers, they represent a loyal audience hungry for the opportunity to develop high levels of skill, to gain control over events, and to feel a sense of belonging to a particular group. Video games offer all this and more, including increased self-respect and the respect of peers. Few children can resist the pull of video games and research has yet to pronounce whether this is a good or bad thing.

The ideas behind computer games

Video games work on many levels, but tend largely to rely on instant gratification. The quality of the music and incidental graphics (backdrops, non-playing images, and so on) is constantly improving on the better games, but there is a steady stream of unimaginative, formulaic products that are indistinguishable from each other. Most games have the same basic components—a static playing area over which moving objects or characters can be controlled. The playing area is usually many times bigger than the screen itself, and different parts scroll on as the player moves to them. Sound effects are very important—studies show that kids playing mute games tire of them much sooner than when the sound is turned on—and serve to give valuable feedback of actions. Some games have so much happening on-screen at once that the player's visual attention has to be concentrated on one small area, despite the fact that important things are happening elsewhere; a successful game gets the mix of peripheral vision and focal point action right, but others are either too visually boring or too complex. The following categories describe the way in which games can be broadly distinguished:

SPORT SIMULATIONS

These are simply electronic versions of popular sports: Golf, tennis, hockey, or athletics. The latest ones include team management, complete tournaments, and considerable background material. It is worth remembering that the very first commercially successful video game, Atari's Pong, was based on ping-pong/tennis, purely because that was the limit of the technology at the time.

RACERS

These are also sports simulations, but concentrate on high speed or performance sports: Formula one racing, motorbike racing, or rough terrain driving.

ADVENTURES

These create fantasy worlds and settings in which the player assumes a role or identity to pursue a series of adventures. Collecting items and tackling the bad guys (by wile as much as violence) are common elements of adventure games.

PUZZLERS

Characters and scenery are less likely to be involved in puzzlers, which are brain teasers or puzzles of shapes, letters, and numbers. Abstract games such as Tetris, Minesweeper, Breakout, and many variants rely on a combination of logic, fast reflexes, split-second coordination, and thinking ahead—this can be potentially addictive.

PLATFORMERS

These are the games that seem to make or break the hardware. Characters run along platforms, jumping over and onto target objects, often with some higher objective (rescuing another character, retrieving a stolen object). Typically, there are puzzles to solve, prizes to collect, and enemies and hazards to avoid or defeat. The pleasure comes from learning how to complete each screen—there may be a prize that seems out of reach until a certain jumping strategy can be attained, or an obstinate enemy that, at first look, just cannot be removed. Nintendo's success in selling consoles was intricately linked with Mario Bros; Sega's, with Sonic the Hedgehog.

PLATFORM BLASTERS

As above, except that characters attempt to blast and destroy everything that appears as they progress along the platform.

BEAT 'EM UPS

These games involve primarily physical violence, when combatants engage in punching, kicking, and throwing. Two players knock each other around using combinations of keys on the game controller and weapons do not figure prominently. Popular examples are Mortal Kombat or Street Fighter, plus any number of spinoffs with increasingly weird combatants.

SHOOT 'EM UPS

As above, except that weapons *do* figure prominently. Characters interact aggressively, shooting and killing an enemy, often extraterrestrial. Space Invaders, Galaxians, and Asteroids are popular targets, each appearing in games which involve a spacecraft or other device moving around and shooting oncoming bad guys, rocks, or both. Twists include having extra arms, ammo, or shields floating past that need some dangerous flying to retrieve, or some enormous mother ship at the end of each level to defeat. This end-of-level treat is often found in many other classes of games.

Many games have elements of more than one of the above categories. Big film tie-ins, such as *Jurassic Park*, will normally absorb part of the plot into an exploratory maze, with combat and platform sequences along the way. More unusually, a game may take a standard theme and exploit it in new ways—there is currently a trend for multi-player platform games, for example, such as Sonic 3. Other interesting new developments are appearing all the time, with film companies contributing many minutes (sometimes hours) of live footage for large exploratory games on CD-ROM based machines. On the wilder shores of gaming, interactive multi-player flight simulators and MUDs (multi-user dungeons) run on large computers with multiple dial-up lines or access links to the Internet, a global computer network providing a shared environment for many serious games.

Video games and addiction

Few people, no matter how disapproving of video games, can shrug them off without a second glance after the first attempt. Video games are powerfully addictive and their compulsive effects can be felt almost immediately, to the extent that addiction is often the most immediate and severe effect of game playing. The term is used with the same meaning to describe the same symptoms of addiction to drugs or alcohol—a compulsive behavioral involvement, a lack of interest in other activities, association mainly with other addicts, and uncomfortable physical and mental symptoms when trying to stop the behavior. What is it about video games that makes them so addictive?

There are two components of addiction: The design of the games themselves, and the psychological characteristics of the players involved with them. At the most basic level, games hook players by rewarding success in a simple stimulus-response cycle. Points are awarded for certain actions, and when more points are awarded for a different type of action, the player immediately wants to repeat the action in an effort to repeat the reward. Interest is sustained by a carefully balanced mixture of frustration, incentive, and reward, allowing new players to build skills gradually and ensuring that they continue to *want* to build greater skills. Better skill means more points, a higher level of game play, and progress into another level of the game, where incidental rewards include new scenery, new hazards, and tougher enemies. Neither consistent rewards nor persistent frustration hook a player so quickly or so firmly as unpredictable rewards. This principle has been demonstrated vividly in animals, who persist in a certain type of behavior for far longer when they cannot predict precisely what will yield a reward. Thus games build up expectations of their players one level at a time, adding different twists and tricks at each level. At all times, it is essential that players are able at least to begin to tackle a problem so that they don't give up, but on the other hand, it cannot be so easy that it loses the element of challenge.

Games also provide far higher levels of stimulation than the real world. Apart from the richly colored fantasy landscapes, games incorporate much greater visual, aural, and mental stimulation, with detailed action sequences beginning any moment. The player is constantly required to think, observe, respond, and perform, call on all sorts of cognitive and coordinating skills to do so. Settings can be local cities or outer space, enchanted forest or eerie swamp, subterranean cavern or distant planet; characters may be human, animal, alien—or indescribable. Success can win anything from the hand of the princess to the salvation of the entire galaxy. Compared to such lavish environments, the reality of being a schoolchild in a small bedroom with homework, rain, and non-combatant interaction can seem desperately dull.

Addiction also arises out of the personality characteristics of the players—although these characteristics are present to a greater or lesser degree in all of us. Some researchers argue that games actually compensate for poor imagination, crushing an individual's own imaginative efforts and hooking in those people who are unable to develop their own daydreams and fantasies to a manageable level. Others suggest that the direct effect of game play on arousal levels provides a pleasurable chemical change in brain chemistry: Some games can "pep you up" while others might have a tranquilizing effect. More recent studies distinguish between two levels of addiction: Primary, describing a direct addiction to games as a test of skill, source of arousal and excitement, and a means of gaining peer respect; and secondary, where the game represents a form of escape from some other, deeper problem, so that play often decreases when the other problem is resolved. Escapist addiction matches closely with images of the awkward loner, although it is not always this severe. Game playing can be a displacement activity while other problems are actually being tackled on a different unconscious level—authors playing Minesweeper while struggling to complete a chapter will know all about this.

Emotional development

The most highly charged debate on video games centers around their effect on children's levels of aggression. Concern stems from the high levels of aggressive conflict which are a theme of many best-selling games, where often the only resolution to a difficulty is to "kill" your electronic opponent. The main issues are almost identical to those surrounding violent films and television shows over the past two or three decades, where the main argument was that repeated exposure to violent films increases aggressive behavior in viewers. Although the film and television debate has not yet been entirely laid to rest, fewer and fewer researchers now subscribe to the opposing view that watching aggressive films can be an outlet for aggression, *reducing* actual expressed violence. Instead, the evidence accumulated over the years has shown more and more overwhelmingly that violent films *do* encourage aggressive behavior in their viewers. The link is not as straightforward as once supposed, however; film-related aggression is rarely a direct replication of observed violence. Instead, repeated viewing of violent films seems to have a gradual "brutalizing" effect. Initial reactions of shock and disgust are gradually replaced with a more tolerant and accepting view: The more violence is repeated, the more acceptable it becomes. When violent acts are performed by a character who is admired or perceived to be the "hero," the rate at which aggression permeates into children's behavior accelerates. If children are no longer shocked or appalled by violent acts, they are more likely to believe violence to be an acceptable means of expressing frustration or resolving disputes. Similarly, others around them are less likely to interfere or express disapproval of an act which has become more widely accepted as "normal" or socially acceptable.

Many popular video games rely on themes of violence and destruction for their appeal, often becoming more and more graphic in their depiction of blood, death, and gore in an effort to win and retain new customers. The key difference between video games and television or film is that video games are interactive, requiring children to engage in the combat in a more active, structured way. Higher levels of on-screen aggression, for example, may serve as a means of achieving the next level in a particular game. It may not even be the content of a game which aggravates the aggressive response: Video games demand skills which take time to learn; before they are fully acquired, the experience can be frustrating and disappointing; both conditions are known to figure in subsequent aggression.

The real effects of prolonged playing with violent, interactive video games are not well known or understood—primarily because the games have not been around for long enough. Nonetheless, existing studies conducted in both the United States and The United Kingdom are beginning to suggest that, like violent films, violent video games increase aggressive behavior in children. The effects are not clear and some are even contradictory, but a majority of studies *does* confirm some correlation between interaction with violent video games and increased aggressive behavior. What is lacking from the current research is any indication of the depth and permanence of these effects. Most were conducted over a relatively short period, with children observed immediately after interacting with the games. A week, month, or year later it is likely that other influences would give rise to different observations.

One factor that does appear to influence children's response to video games is their inherent personality type, particularly the Type A and Type B traits discussed in Chapter 1 in the context of stress. Children with Type A personality characteristics (perfectionism, obsession with punctuality, high need for achievement) seem to be more likely to respond aggressively than do their more easygoing Type B peers. They are also slightly more likely to experience depression and anxiety as a result of doing badly in computerized battles against either a human or electronic component. If personality variables can influence the aggressive response, it seems likely that other variables will also have an effect. These could be factors like family background, extent and quality of social relationships, even progress at school.

Whatever the unknowns of video games and violence (and there are many), it is impossible to dismiss games as a factor in increased levels of violent and aggressive behavior. Best-sellers such as Doom II and Quake, which focus entirely on gruesome fights-to-the-death, typically presented as glamorous acts of heroism, are unlikely to persuade children of the virtues of pacifism. It remains to be seen, however, what the deeper, long-term effects of video game playing are likely to be. The only indication we have to date is that of television and the effect of violent films. Although the debate is unresolved, it is now largely accepted that long-term exposure to violent films does make violent behavior seem more normal and more appropriate to certain people.

On the positive side, the very best-selling video games are not violent—neither Super Mario Brothers nor Sonic the Hedgehog involves any blood or death at all. Even "shoot 'em ups" are not necessarily bloodthirsty. Many involve nothing more than anonymous objects (home spaceships versus alien spaceships, for example) blasting one another without necessarily requiring ghoulish graphics or sound effects. When an invader is shot, it simply disappears instead of falling bleeding to the floor, which removes the worrisome realism which a small but growing number of violent games now include. Even so, the number of games featuring realistic murder and mutilation is increasing, the primary goal being increased sales to an older and more affluent audience who demand this type of material. This has prompted calls for certification of video games to provide guidance for parents and buyers. While this is clearly a good idea, it raises the uncomfortable issues of game desirability—games which receive an X-rating will immediately become the most highly sought after.

Social development

Violent or not, video games can preoccupy children to the exclusion of all else, keeping them glued to the screen for hours on end. Irrespective of the content of the game, this cannot be healthy, and the possibility of damaged social development is another worrying side-effect.

Normal social development takes place as a result of long-term interaction with other people. Parents pass on to their children basic values and codes of right and wrong, with which they are then equipped to meet the outside world. The full process of socialization takes place over years, as children learn to cope with the needs and wishes of others through interaction with teachers, friends, and peers. During this process, they acquire self-control, the capacity to share, and the ability to work as part of a team. They learn the importance of taking turns, to give and accept criticism, initiate and sustain friendships. They begin to recognize different emotions in different people and develop an ability to empathize—understand how others may feel about an event or person which does not affect the child directly. Ultimately, the process of socialization prepares children for long-term, mature relationships in both a personal and professional capacity.

The school years are clearly crucial to children's successful socialization, with classroom, sports, and club meetings providing the diversity of settings and activities which teach vital life skills. Computer and video games are now an integral element of school life and, as such, are going to have an impact on the socialization process. Unlike many sports and activities (cycling, roller-skating, or football, for example), video games are not active (in the physical sense). They do not require children to develop their imagination, since video worlds are already rich in fantasy. Many do not require the presence of another person—children can play against the computer—and none requires children to leave their bedrooms. The implication is that game playing can prevent children from acquiring and developing the social and life skills so essential to their future happiness and stability, turning them instead into awkward, isolated individuals caught up in a fantasy world. One experiment on the effects of game play on socialization had children of varying ages play either aggressive or "friendly" games. Afterwards, younger children were, on the whole, less willing to share sweets and toys than older children, and children who played aggressive video games were far less willing to share than those who played the friendly games. This suggests that, although playing the nonviolent video game did not increase sharing behavior, playing the aggressive video game tended to suppress this behavior, more so in younger children.

As with the debate on violence, it is still too early to say with any confidence that video games do or do not have a damaging effect on social development. Early research shows that dedicated gamers have a tendency to anthropomorphize their computers, attributing human characteristics to them and treating them as "friends." How harmful this may be is unclear—many people give their cars names and personalities with no adverse consequences—but it can become alarming if taken to extremes. It may also be worth noting that (unlike anthropomorphic drivers) gamers almost never attribute female personalities to their computers. Children may come to prefer the company of their computers to that of human friends, since the machine's behavior is more predictable, more controllable, and less demanding. There are even programs available which give a "personality" to the computer, prompting it to "chat" to its user at random moments, even enabling it to "learn" more about a person from the answers given.

Games enthusiasts argue that games actually encourage teamwork, and in many cases this appears to be true. A large number of games are designed for two or more players, and some of the larger and more sophisticated creations operate across entire networks which can be accessed by many players at a time. The benefits of such multiple playing will only be apparent where cooperation is required of the characters, however. In many instances, players are better served by looking after themselves and treating every other player as an enemy. Games for two players encourage a similarly selfish, competitive outlook—while it is important to learn your opponent's strategy and skills, the overriding aim is to destroy him. "Team" games may encourage children to get together, but whether they teach team skills seems more doubtful.

Intellectual development

Less clear is the effect of video games playing on intellectual development, since there is evidence that certain types of interaction can be beneficial in many ways. Before drawing any conclusions about intellectual development, it is important to be aware that certain children are more likely to have access to video and computer games. Both the hardware and software necessary for gaming are expensive, so regular game players tend to come from better-off families who are able to support the habit. Gamers are also more likely to have regular access to a computer, either at home or at school, than their non-playing friends (although this doesn't apply so widely to users of the Nintendo and Sega consoles, which plug into the television). Hand-held consoles are also more readily available, but offer a narrower range of games. What this means is that regular gamers are more likely to have general access to computers and are more likely to be from affluent families. Such children will therefore begin their gaming careers with the advantages these circumstances convey—greater familiarity with technology, more stable family environment, and better educational resources. Any findings with regard to intellectual development should be considered in this context.

The nature of many software applications makes them ideal for educational purposes, where constant interaction can occur between child and learning material. Interactive learning is known to "fix" new knowledge more quickly and deeply than passive rote learning, opening up a vast potential for games which also include an educational element. Few games make any pretensions to be educational, however, and yet still claim additional cognitive benefits. Citing the rapid, stimulating interaction as a source of benefits, manufacturers suggest that gaming improves hand-eye coordination, encourages greater exploratory behavior and greater initiative. Constant demands to solve electronic problems and tackle aggressors lead a child to think, plan, and develop strategies; these are cognitive functions which, manufacturers argue, transfer readily into educational and life situations. That games require these skills is certain; what is less clear is how well they transfer into other thinking modes, or even whether the skills acquired are relevant to any real-life situation. Many "skills" are not the problem-solving kind but simply keyboard skills; and the development of a strategy to get Aladdin across a field of burning coals will not readily transfer into a strategy for planning other activities or meeting real life goals. Claims that gaming introduces children to computer technology are no less tenuous: Children who play games already have access to and familiarity with the technology, and there is little relation between gaming software and the office automation applications discussed elsewhere in this book.

More hopefully, there is a small number of games which sacrifice profit-generating violence for more constructive activity, in some cases almost as lucrative. The popular SimCity (for "simulation") requires players to construct and manage a fictitious city, balancing housing versus business development, planning parks and shopping centers, dealing with social issues such as crime, unemployment, and pollution, and tackling natural disasters such as earthquakes and fires. As in the real world, simulated civic harmony is a question of balance and trade-offs. Intensive business development will reduce unemployment but increase pollution and the demand for housing; large parks and shopping centers cost money. Simplistic solutions to problems, such as raising taxes to fund new developments, can result in a net outflow of the population; and natural disasters can strike at any time. SimCity teaches children the "opportunity-cost" of every decision and the importance of planning and balance. Although a relatively simplified representation of the world, the action in SimCity does show how complex apparently simple decisions can be; and it does demonstrate the large number of factors which influence and are influenced by such decisions. Such lessons are undoubtedly valuable for real situations, and if a child learns no more than that a link might exist between crime and unemployment, the seeds are sown for deeper thought in later life.

Sex differences in computing: Stereotypes and political incorrectness

With many organizations making deliberate efforts to recruit and train more women into computing, it is important for girls to be encouraged from an early age to become more involved in technology. Although computer and video games appear to represent an ideal opportunity for this sort of spontaneous exploration, there are fears that computers are becoming "masculinized" at a far earlier stage than ever before. Boys appear to be dominating game play, alienating their sisters from computers before they even understand what they can do.

The love of technology for technology's sake—gadgets—seems to be a peculiarly male phenomenon. From wristwatches to hi-fi systems to cameras to cars, if it has buttons, knobs, dials, and displays it will be a male object of desire. Women remain indifferent to a car which can reach 150 mph when the speed limit is 70 mph; to a man, such a machine is greatly preferable to one which can only manage a paltry 120 mph. These sex differences seem fairly universal, the most blunt conclusion being that men like technology for technology's sake; women like it only if it can really do something for them. There is no clear explanation for this. Some researchers trace it back to our primitive roots, suggesting that Woman the Homemaker learned to focus only on genuinely useful implements in her quest for safety and thrift in the home; some cite patterns of brain development, showing that the right hemisphere of the brain (controlling abstract and spatial reasoning) is better developed in men, whereas the logical, analytical left hemisphere dominates in more reason. Others believe it is a more recent phenomenon, the result of socialization which keeps women away from science and technology and drives them instead into artistic and domestic pursuits.

There is plenty of research to show that women *use* computers whereas men *love* them. The difference is important: Women are more likely to acquire specific, relevant, and productivity-oriented skills, while men dabble in whatever they can find. Women are prompt about asking for help when problems occur, while men prefer to solve it themselves, however long it takes. The result is women who get the job done quickly, knowing only what they need to know; and men who attain a broad technical knowledge which is rarely goal-oriented. It is difficult to say which is better—ideally, a combination of both. While men tend to eschew the rational perception of computers as a tool for achieving more important goals, women rarely acquire the confidence and experience to make innovative leaps of exploration. The result is a markedly higher proportion of women than men displaying "computerphobia," an inexplicably negative and hostile attitude towards computing. The rare individuals who are able to combine the confidence to explore new technology with an awareness of how their skills can contribute to real-life problems tend to be extremely successful in the computing industry.

Whatever the relative merits of male and female approaches to computers, the long-term effect seems likely to work against women. It all begins in childhood, with children's relationships to computer and video games. Even without computer games to play, girls and boys tend to spend their leisure time very differently: Girls like to have a broad range of interests—talking to friends, reading, shopping, and getting involved in after-school activities. Boys tend to stick with a single hobby, maybe collecting football cards or playing video games. Girls are more likely to describe video games as "pointless" or "boring" and are better at resisting the addictive elements of gaming. While this does broaden the social skills of girls, it also deprives them of valuable opportunities to learn about the basic capabilities of technology and acquire the confidence for more profitable exploration in later life.

There is a gender-related difference between male and female cognitive skills, some of which are particularly pertinent to video game play. Boys tend to have better depth perception and spatial reasoning skills (related to greater specialization of the right hemisphere of the brain) which makes them better able to navigate around an electronic landscape. Girls, with greater left hemisphere specialization, are better at analytical games, tending to outperform boys on puzzlers, particularly those of a verbal nature. Although these differences occur naturally, they need not have a permanent effect on children's lives. The young brain is remarkably flexible, and practice will certainly improve cognitive skills even if they are not dominant to begin with. This does not seem to be happening, however—both Sega and Nintendo have marketed games specifically aimed at girls; both have failed. Instead, girls shun active participation and seem to prefer a supportive or "cheerleader" role while brothers and boyfriends demonstrate their skills, While inherent sex differences change the way girls and boys relate to computers, there are other elements which reinforce these patterns.

Violent elements particularly are more likely to turn girls away from video games, a fact which already seems to be fueling a cycle of electronic sexist violence. The feedback loop between male players (and buyers) and male developers is skewing the nature of the games towards more violence, increasingly directed at female characters. Where females are not portrayed as the victims of the player's violent male character, they turn up as the quiveringly helpless victims of other male bad guys within the game, unable to do much beyond wait to be rescued. Such games give male players far greater power over electronic females; and this persists into adult games where sexually submissive females encourage male characters to initiate aggressive sexual encounters. The fear is clearly that such stereotypes encourage players (both male and female) to transfer their expectations of male and female behavior from the screen to the real world, reinforcing archaic and dangerous notions of violent male dominance at a very early age. Again, it is too early to say how true this is; today's gamers are the first generation to be exposed to such a phenomenon and are not yet old enough to be displaying the effects.

What the Game Boys say: Sega and Nintendo

Many of the issues associated with video and computer game play are controversial in the extreme, dealing as they do with the impressionable minds of young children. The two most successful manufacturers of this market are Sega and Nintendo, both Japanese, both overnight multi-million dollar companies, both vying for the hearts of young players with the kind of intensity to be found in their video games. Both organizations express due concern for parental fears of antisocial behavior and mind-warping aggression, but both are also sinking immense resources into identifying what makes children buy (or persuade their parents to buy) games, and are catering to these factors in their marketing. The most successful vendors are acutely aware of children's passion for "street culture" and their delight in anything their parents hate.

At the time of writing, Sega appears to have an open mind about medical research into epilepsy and short-sightedness, and feels that parents should decide what games are appropriate and monitor children's playing hours. The company says that it has offered a large amount of cash to fund research into children's health, but that "no one seems to have shown any interest in following it up." Nintendo has a much clearer set of guidelines for game content and is prepared to comment on the issues parents worry about. The company has produced a leaflet: *The Ninfinite World of Video Games—what you never dared to ask: A Parent's Guide*. It is brief and glossy but does deal with questions of aggression, social isolation, and education, emphasizing the need for balance and parental supervision. Nintendo also bans the use of sexual and sexist language and imagery in its games, as well as excessive violence, domestic violence, racist and religious slurs, the use of drugs and alcohol, excessive force, and political messages.

While it is heartening to see influential organizations taking a responsible attitude to their customers, it is important to remember the large number of other, smaller companies with less strict ethical attitudes. It is also true that none of these companies is in it for the good of their health (or anyone else's for that matter). Games manufacturers are profit-driven corporations who want to make money, and all else is secondary. It may take external or legislative influence to identify the best practices for games design and see that it is followed.

Medical problems

While their parents wrestle with repetitive strain injuries, stress, and boredom, children have a whole new set of computer-related medical problems to contend with.

EPILEPSY

Fears that games induce epilepsy in previously healthy children are largely groundless, although there is more controversial research surrounding the effects of games as a trigger for more frequent attacks in children who already suffer from the condition. Epilepsy is a neurological condition in which the normal activity of the brain becomes disrupted. Messages become garbled, resulting in either full-scale *grand mal* tonic-clonic seizures, or briefer *petit mal* minor seizures. In the former, patients may black out, their bodies may jerk or twitch and they may froth at the mouth and cry out. Minor seizures involve altered vision, muscle twitching, or mental confusion, or even split-second blackouts.

A proportion of people who have epilepsy (around five to ten percent) are photosensitive—that is, susceptible to flashing lights and light patterns. Both natural and flickering light can precipitate the seizures, but the most common appears to be television or stroboscopic lights, often used at discos. In the U.S., television usually works at 60 Hz, that is, an image repetition rate of sixty times per second. This frequency can trigger fits in less than 40 percent of photosensitive people, regardless of content. Lower rates of repetition are more dangerous: An old or badly adjusted TV, flickering at 25 hertz, could cause problems for a child close to it. By contrast, children using a hand-held console or modern TV with a remote control are far less likely to be at risk. The console offers a small screen in the middle of a visual field with other things happening on the periphery, and its LCD technology means there is no repetition cycle over and over.

Part of the problem in drawing firm conclusions is the age of game players and onset of seizures. It is common for people with epilepsy to experience their first seizure during adolescence, any time between the ages of ten and twenty. This matches closely with the age range targeted by Sega and Nintendo. Nintendo has taken the issue seriously and, at the time of writing, is funding and carrying out a full-scale study into the phenomenon in partnership with Sega. These intentions are laudable, but it is nevertheless a little discomfiting to know that the money funding the research will be coming from an organization with a lot at stake if it gets an answer it does not like. To help in resolving the matter, the United Kingdom's Department of Trade and Industry commissioned the National Epilepsy Society to study the alleged link between computer games and epilepsy in a report published in December 1993. The study was launched in May 1993 after several cases of epilepsy among young players of video games, but found no evidence that photosensitivity itself can be caused by playing video games, watching TV, or by other light sources. Photosensitive individuals are more vulnerable to the effects of these light sources than their nonphotosensitive friends, but computer games are no more likely to trigger epileptic seizures than television. With this limited knowledge, both Sega and Nintendo have opted to include information leaflets and guidelines with each game sold. Current research on epilepsy is not entirely adequate, but certainly points the finger of blame away from computer games.

Current medical advice for parents of photosensitive children who have epilepsy is straightforward. Children are safest with a hand-held LCD console, but will be almost as safe if the television is modern and has a remote control (avoiding the need to get up close). Children using TVs to play should sit well back from the screen—at least ten feet—and the room should be well lit. Computer screens generally have too high a refresh rate (see pp. 16-17) to induce epilepsy, but it is still advisable to reduce contrast levels and discourage children from peering too closely at the screen. Whatever this may mean for those who have epilepsy, it will certainly help reduce eyestrain and headaches. Lack of sleep and unrelated worries can aggravate photosensitivity, so don't let tired children play games, and try to enforce regular breaks—hourly ideally. Children who are known to be photosensitive can be helped by wearing an eye patch—images of flickering light are processed more haphazardly when both eyes are watching, so if one eye is covered the chances of flicker triggering a seizure are reduced.

REPETITIVE STRAIN INJURY

Even children can suffer from RSI, although it is a slightly different type from that encountered by the adult computer-using population. In most cases, the symptoms are similar to those of more conventional RSI, but the areas afflicted are different. Because of the intensive keyboard and joystick action required for some computer games, children have been known to develop the aptly named "Nintendonitis," pain and inflammation of the tendons, particularly those of the thumb and forefinger. Related conditions include "Pac-Man's elbow" and "Space Invader's revenge," various skin, joint, and muscle complaints related to prolonged and intensive game play. Other minor conditions may be blisters, calluses, and temporary numbness of the hand and lower arm. The important difference between video-game and work-related RSI is that game-related conditions lack the complex social roots that affect adults. Children are not required by the terms of any contract to play games, nor must they achieve known goals within a time limit. Children play games because they want to and choose to, and this eliminates all the hard-to-quantify factors which play such an important but intangible role in the more serious and prolonged diseases of adulthood. In this case, it is possible to treat children's RSI with simpler measures such as rest and increased variety of leisure pursuits.

SHORT-SIGHTEDNESS

Does staring at a screen for hours on end induce short-sightedness in children? Although the intuitive answer is "yes," the true answer is far less clear cut—many believe it to be "no." Eyes are as susceptible as any other part of the body to fatigue when overused, and children who never take a break from their consoles and computers will invariably experience the soreness, dryness, and grittiness their hard-working parents suffer from. The evidence is confusing. On the one hand, it is undoubtedly true that literate societies have significantly more short-sighted individuals than do illiterate societies, providing strong evidence for a link between close visual work and myopia. In support of this, children with glasses at an early age may well be tested, but they also tend to acquire a reputation for being "brainy." On the other hand, there are plenty of people who read widely and don't require glasses, while non-readers peer myopically from an early age. Children tend to have stronger visual function and can tense and relax the lens more quickly than adults, so they should be more resistant to eyestrain. Some children are born with marked visual defects which actually improve as they grow older.

With little apparent causality, some researchers argue that short-sightedness is genetically determined to the same extent that, say, intelligence or verbal skill is. It is possible, in that case, that the *genes* for short-sightedness and an early ability to read are linked in some way—more literate children are likely to be short-sighted too, not because one causes the other but because the genes which control the two tendencies often occur together. Over the years, this could make for a genetic pooling of myopics, since people of similar background and education tend to marry, concentrating the genes controlling short-sightedness in a smaller population. It is certainly a plausible theory and could explain otherwise random links between game-play and myopia, but with no evidence yet for a gene controlling myopia, it is hard to make it stick.

As discussed in Chapter 5, it is safe to assume only that prolonged game-play can aggravate visual problems which are already there, but is unlikely actually to cause short-sightedness. To that end, it is equally safe to recommend eye care techniques such as regular breaks, good, well-balanced lighting, minimal contrast, and sitting well back from the screen. Children should also receive regular eye tests from a qualified optometrist to ensure that any latent problems are identified and treated early.

PHYSICAL FITNESS

There has been a lot of concern expressed in recent years about the declining fitness among young people, particularly children. A vast range of factors is involved here, but computers and video game-playing must take their share of the blame. Nutritional factors are widely implicated, but worries are largely centered on children who spurn outdoor exercise in favor of television-watching and computer game-playing. Days in the classroom and evenings and weekends at the computer are turning children into one of the most sedentary groups in the population, with fitness levels well below that which doctors consider acceptable or safe. While it will not do children any immediate harm to be unfit, it does lay patterns for problems in later life, some of which can be severe. People who never attain reasonable fitness will find it increasingly difficult to achieve and maintain any sort of fitness as they grow older, and poor health habits in children (particularly boys) lead directly to an increased risk of heart disease later on.

Many people are quite happy to let children stay indoors with their computers, for whole weekends at a time in some cases. It keeps them off the streets, parents know where they are and feel comfortable that they are safe inside. All this is true, but it is also true that children are losing precious time required to build fitness and (if they are alone) make friends and learn social skills. It is definitely worth encouraging children to become more involved in team sports and after-school sport activities as an antidote to intensive computing and gaming sessions. This way, children receive supervision, remain in a safe, known location, and learn the fitness and people skills they need now and as they grow up.

Educational and "edutainment" software

It became clear relatively early on in the development of the personal computer that here was a machine which could facilitate learning. Based purely on its numerical abilities, the least a computer can do is serve as a big calculator. Used more thoughtfully, it can be used in an interactive math lesson, play a part in the teaching of programming (and the processes of logical thought, planning, and goal-setting which that implies), and manipulate letters and words.

It is here, in the realms of educational software, that real hope lies for the computer and its relationship to children. Not simply because educational software is good for kids and that makes parents happy, nor because of the total absence of blood and severed heads (although this helps). Educational software—now dubbed "edutainment" software—is the way forward because it can combine (with breathtaking ease) enough fun and stimulation to keep children happy, amused, and interested for hours, with new knowledge in a richer and deeper format than any book. Many people shrug off educational software as a series of computerized textbooks—a little more flashy but basically just as boring—and traditionally this has been true, at least in part. The development of educational software has been slow because the obvious customers—schools—have never had the money to justify corporations sinking big-time resources into this area. All this is changing with the advent of multimedia—a dream environment for educationalists—and a new discerning parental customer, demanding something more constructive than Streetfighter II for his or her youngster.

Multimedia has brought two crucial elements to the education market: Sound, and far greater capacity, usually in the form of CD-ROM. The result is a generation of programs which can pack in huge amounts of material to interact with children far more closely. Equipped with a sound card, the computer can read words for children too young to read themselves; with the resources of a CD-ROM drive, there is room to allow rich color and animation, and the creation of talking characters which escort children through stories and puzzles. From simple spelling tasks where the computer "speaks" a word and the child types it, to the lavish *Encyclopedia Britannica* which leads children through a fabulously comprehensive electronic book of cross-referenced facts, to more complex and recent innovations, software which educates as it entertains is where the richest imaginations and more thoughtful developers seem to be gathering.

The complexity and sheer size that multimedia makes possible have made it easier to make better software. The diversity is amazing—software can now teach children history, geography, spelling, numerical and spatial reasoning, biology, chemistry, physics, and astronomy, all without the child resisting. In most "edutainment" products, the learning is incidental to the main objective—often to find a missing object or person, and traveling through time, space, and the planet to do so. Little suspecting that their voyages are designed to teach, children derive the same pleasure from sneakily "stopping-off" en route to learn about The Cherokee Nation or Moscow in the nineteenth century, for example, that they previously did from reading comics beneath the desk during math lessons. Without the pressure to "pay attention!" to lessons which instantly become boring, children can become tremendously absorbed in new, interactive information which teaches them at least as much as a lesson. And there are more people than programmers at work on edutainment software: Today's packages adhere faithfully to psychological principles of child development and education. Children are rewarded for getting something right and never blamed for getting it wrong. They are given endless opportunities to return to a difficult word or concept without being made to feel they are holding things up, and they are talked to in a way which matches their own language levels.

Edutainment software works best for children between the ages of four and twelve, although there is certainly enough material in many of them to keep even well-educated adults on their toes. For older children who have acquired a taste for learning, such games can teach valuable research skills: The ease with which you can switch from one "page" to another to follow upon a new idea shows children the importance of understanding all the components of a particular item of knowledge, and the ways to pursue it. The one danger with such products is that parents may be tempted to relinquish all involvement in their child's progress, leaving them instead to the patient, untiring efforts of the computer. Whatever children may learn from thoughtful, well-designed software, there are still no computers which can provide the benefits they receive from regular, frequent parental involvement in their progress—and that means knowing when it is time to stop absorbing and start applying.

Managing children's computing time

Every new technology has its downside, and the uncontrolled spread of new "unsuitable" computer games is certainly one of the most worrisome aspects of computing technology. Parents are faced with the choice of either banning computers (impossible and inappropriate), hoping they don't do any harm (irresponsible), or attempting to stay one step ahead of them (equally impossible).

Sadly, there is little you can do to force children away from their computers, but the following points may help:

- Don't break addiction by banning the child from using the computer—it will probably fuel the urge to play.
- Negotiate allowed and forbidden times to play, and stick to them.
- During "forbidden" times, organize other activities for children. Go out for day trips, take children shopping, or get them involved in other, more active hobbies.
- Encourage friendships with children who themselves pursue active, non-computer-related hobbies. Peer pressure can exert a powerful influence.
- If desperate, there are electronic blocking devices which can prevent the television from being used during specified periods. It is also possible to buy locks for computer hard disks and CD-ROM drives, but make sure children know when access will be denied.
- Finally, don't become over anxious about game-playing or get into conflict with "hooked" kids Even if children get bored with a game, the knowledge that their parents hate it will persuade them to keep on playing. Like many normal stages of childhood, the fascination with computer games can disappear as suddenly and mysteriously as it appeared.

CHAPTER 8

Computers, Health, and the Law

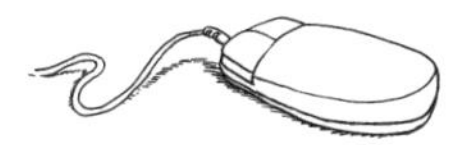

THE QUESTION OF LEGISLATION for computer-related health and safety is not a simple one. While it is intuitively good to have laws which protect our health during work, in practice this is extraordinarily difficult to implement. As this book has tried to show, the many issues which affect health in relation to the computer are far from clear-cut, and much of the law relies on precise definitions of those issues with which it deals. Planning, writing, and clarifying the law which deals with these issues is necessarily problematic, and can lead to vast amounts of unwieldy legislation that cannot realistically be applied in a working environment. To avoid this, the tendency is often to make definitions as general as possible to allow for maximum flexibility.

Although no conclusive evidence has yet emerged to suggest that computer users are vulnerable to serious health threats, there is plenty of evidence for general and sometimes prolonged health problems if computing equipment is not used correctly, or used within a harmful environment.

What the legislation says

The point of legislation is clearly to protect the health of employees within the working environment. It is not, as many companies fear, an exercise intended to impose impractical and expensive demands on tight budgets; nor is it a series of inflexible requirements which demand highly specific steps to be taken. Quite the reverse, in fact—many of the requirements are couched in somewhat vague terms, but this does not represent any lack of precision on the part of the legislators, rather, it is an attempt to provide employers with the flexibility to impose elements of their own interpretation on *potentially* expensive legal requirements. Thus the use of terms such as "suitable" and "appropriate" (when referring to screen flicker, for example) are used to imply that no absolute or measurable standard exists and that a company's final choice of flicker level can legitimately be determined by the general consensus of employees rather than any hard-and-fast rule. Recommendations of what is likely to be regarded as "appropriate" by a majority of people are generally supplied in such examples.

Terms and definitions

Legal documents are, by their very nature, complex and protracted, designed by lawyers to be read by other lawyers and rarely comprehensible to the layperson. This is not a deliberate policy (although it often seems so at the time), but a means of ensuring a minimum of ambiguities (and therefore loopholes) if it ever comes to court action over some aspect of any given law. The exercise of defining terms and clarifying statements often takes up more paper than the legislation itself. To begin with, therefore, it is important to define the scope of the legislation and the people and equipment it really effects. Its purpose is to make employers responsible for the health and safety of their computer-using employees, and the target of the legislation is the *user* in the context of his or her *workstation*, where *display screen equipment* is used. Knowing what these terms refer to is half the battle:

THE USER

Not merely an employee, the user is "anyone who habitually uses display screen equipment as a significant part of his or her work." Critically, "users" are people who require a computer to do their jobs properly or are required by their employer to use one. The law applies equally to employees who work at home, as long as they are working for a given employer. Clearly, words such as "habitually" and "significant" have no precise meaning and are subject to interpretation. A "habitual user" could be thought of as someone who uses a computer regularly, probably daily, for periods of an hour or more; a person whose work requires weekly, intense stints of computer work; or a home-based worker processing data in batches in his or her own time. It is unwise to impose strict definitions on the term "user" since this increases the number of exceptions—most people will have some feeling about whether or not they consider themselves to be a "user" and, where possible, it is better to play safe.

DISPLAY SCREEN EQUIPMENT

Any alphanumeric or graphic display, be it cathode ray tube, liquid crystal, or other new or emerging technology, counts as display screen equipment. Television and film screens are not included, unless they are used primarily to display text, numbers, or graphics.

WORKSTATION

The legislation affects users in the context of their "immediate work environment"—the workstation. The term includes display screen equipment and also the keyboard, software, other input devices and peripherals, as well as the desk, chair, telephone, and work surfaces. The term "environment" can be safely taken to mean air quality, lighting, and noise, since these are integral to an employee's health and welfare.

Who's responsible for what?

Responsibility for the bulk of the action lies with employers, although employees and manufacturers are expected to play their part, too.

Employers are responsible for performing "an analysis of workstations in order to evaluate the safety and health condition to which they give rise," and are subsequently required to "take appropriate measures to remedy the risks found on the basis of the evaluation." Their responsibilities also include ensuring that minimum standards are applied to all components of the workstation; keeping themselves and their employees informed of related developments; providing training to all employees in the use of workstation components; and ensuring that all employees take regular breaks or changes of activity to reduce or break up the amount of time spent at the workstation. Employers are also obliged to provide regular eye tests for workstation users (on request), and will have to pay for glasses or other "corrective appliances appropriate for the work concerned," provided such appliances are required primarily to make computer use possible.

Employees are responsible for using workstations and related equipment "correctly"—that is, according to the training which their employer should provide. They are also expected to bring problems to the attention of their employer immediately and to cooperate in the correction of these problems.

Manufacturers are required to ensure that their products comply with current standards and, in the interests of survival, almost all the major manufacturers already fulfill the minimum requirements and have done so for several years. This is done by maintaining compliance with one or more standards, and these are discussed in more detail in the following pages.

Who can afford to ignore the regulations?

Not many people. The legislation came into force immediately for organizations planning to buy new workstations or other computing products and has been active since December 1992, where workstations were used for the first time or altered after this date. To every law, however, there are exclusions and this is no exception. No part of the regulations applies to computer systems on board any kind of transport, nor to computers intended for public use, cash tills, typewriters of any description, or portable computers—so long as they are not being used as desktop machines at the workstation.

What the law really means

So much for the legalese—but what does it all mean? The bottom line is that employers are now directly responsible for the health and safety of their employees, specifically, in this case, of employees who use computers as part of their job. They are obliged to demonstrate this responsibility by carrying out a formal evaluation of the working environment and acting on any feedback from the evaluation. Any shortcomings must be corrected, and workers must be consulted where changes are going to affect them. It seems like a tall order—but there is a great deal more to gain than there is to lose.

The evaluation is the vital starting point of an ergonomic overhaul. This should be done either by an employee recognized as competent, or an independent professional ergonomist, and will cover workplace design, including computer hardware, lighting, cooling, humidity, and software. A number of consultancies are able to provide this type of ergonomic audit and some provide awareness seminars to increase awareness of the legislation and its implications. Where they are available it is sensible to attend, since ignorance of the law is no longer acceptable as an excuse for non-compliance.

Practical steps for employers

Before the audit is carried out, perform your own to gain an idea of where problems might be. Ask employees if they are comfortable and if not, encourage them to specify why. Small companies can do this informally, either in face-to-face interviews or at a single meeting, while larger organizations might wish to design a simple questionnaire or check existing assessment tools. Review your computer-buying plans and check with the manufacturers you are interested in that they are aware of current standards and comply with them. Happily, almost all the major manufacturers are acutely aware of the legislation and have complied with it and preceding acts for years—they simply cannot afford not to. Most computer manufacturers are trying to do more to reduce emission levels by complying to standards arrived at independently by research laboratories.

If you want to be sure that radiation is minimized even below acceptable levels, check which standard your potential supplier conforms to. For pregnant women, zero-emission LCD screens are available from some manufacturers, albeit at a price roughly five times greater than that of the standard monitor. Despite its emotive overtones, radiation should not be a major cause for concern among employees.

THE ERGONOMIC AUDIT

The audit is potentially the most daunting step towards compliance, although the closer you get before the audit takes place, the less shocking the outcome. No one will provide free audits, so if you are small and prepared to take the risk, it may be appealing to skip the formal audit altogether and make arrangements based on your own interpretation of the legislation. This might appear to be cheap and satisfactory, but the penalties will be that much higher if an inspector disagrees with your definition of "acceptable." A far better plan is to educate an appointed person in the details of the act, preferably someone with experience with or an interest in health and safety, who can make an accurate judgment about the state of your offices. On the basis of these recommendations, draw up a strategy to overcome obvious problems and then call in the auditors; if you're making an effort, the audit will be quicker and its recommendations cheaper.

FURNITURE AND LIGHTING

The law requires that lighting should be "satisfactory" and provide "an appropriate contrast" between screen and background; this does not mean spending a fortune on hi-tech spotlights. Check that screens are turned away from direct lighting which glares off the screen, and that other light sources are adequate to illuminate paper-based documents. Some people, especially copy typists and others requiring fine visual discrimination, prefer desk lights or spotlights, which is fine so long as they are balanced by more diffuse lighting throughout the office.

As discussed in Chapter 4, research from a number of resources suggests that lighting levels of between 500 and 700 lux (one lux being equivalent to the illumination given off by a standard candle at one meter) are most suitable for an office environment. Strip lights located in the ceiling are generally adequate, as are ceiling spotlights and desk spotlights. Some lights include blinds or faders, and blinds should be present on all windows. Don't panic, however; you are not trying to achieve the intimate lighting of a restaurant or private study in your office, just comfortable, glare-free lighting which enables employees to carry out their jobs without having to squint, peer, don their sunglasses, or shine a flashlight.

Furniture is also perceived as a cash-hungry quagmire which never quite fits the bill. It need not be like this; most furniture designed for office use is adequate. Computer users require comfortable (your definition is as valid as anyone else's) swivel chairs with adjustable seats and backs; they do not need the latest in ergonomic breakthroughs upholstered in leather and including motorized back rest and a lumbar spinal region massage option. Many "ergonomic" items are not ergonomic at all; to qualify for this label, furniture should have received input from a recognized testing professional organization and have been through rigorous testing procedures. Similarly with desks: If a desk is around 27 inches in height and sufficiently wide to accommodate a personal computer and keyboard, it conforms. If this height is too great for shorter people, footrests can be provided for them.

Apart from the radiation issues, look out for other features of your proposed desktop machine. The personal computer you commit yourself to should, of course, include the tilt and swivel features described above; a 15 to 20 degree angle is generally sufficient to ward off the obvious causes of neck and eye strain. Despite the many attractions of the notebook personal computer, you should avoid it as a permanent machine because the integrated keyboard and tiny screen are prime culprits in RSI and neck and eye pain. Look for resolution better than a television (at least 600 by 800)—you should not be able to distinguish dots and lines up close. Keyboards need large, concave keys (½ inch square) which limit the movement on your wrists. Symbols and characters on the keys should be clear and should contrast with the background color of the keys; despite the stigma of "large type," larger letters do reduce typing errors. Mice should support the 90 degree arm-to-body angle, and should not be gripped too lightly; mouse pads prevent the frustration caused by an over-polished desk.

Noise pollution might not be something that many offices are familiar with or confident to control. Again, current standards try to accommodate this and do not specify difficult-to-measure decibel levels—it's up to you and your employees to decide what is acceptable and what is distracting. Printers are particularly noisy offenders, but achieving compliance often requires little more than the removal of the printer to a more remote corner of the office via longer cables, or the construction of partitions around it. Heat and humidity are again dependent on what feels good. Optimum levels for alertness and productivity are estimated to be 70 degrees Fahrenheit with 45 to 65 percent humidity, although if your employees are happy with an alternative specification, that's up to them.

SOFTWARE

Something which is overlooked too often in the quest for ergonomic perfection is the quality of software. Ergonomics has a wide scope, encompassing the entire range of environmental factors, including software, which impact upon computer users. To make the point, current standards make a clear statement about the characteristics of acceptable software, with particular reference to the principles which it should observe. Software should be suitable for the task. This means providing a spreadsheet, not a database, where a spreadsheet is called for. Employers are required to analyze the tasks upon which their employees are engaged and to provide software which makes this task easier—again, this requires communication between employer and employee.

Software is also expected to be easy to use, adaptable to the operator's level of experience, able to provide feedback on user performance and to display information which is meaningful to the operator. Software usability is not easy to determine, and the job is made more difficult by the large numbers of competing products which all claim to offer "usability" as a feature. The competitive nature of software design has inhibited establishing usability guidelines, with manufacturers preferring to concentrate on features and functions. Many products are now saturated in underutilized features and pay scant attention to the ease with which users are able to achieve acceptable productivity levels, creating a costly circle of frustration and avoidance on the part of the user. Read Chapter 2 to gain a clearer idea of basic usability principles for choosing software.

Look for products which show genuine concern for user needs—carefully constructed dialogue boxes, thoughtful on-line help, appropriate use of graphics, and friendly feedback on user actions. Ask to see demonstrations of short-listed products and get staff to test them out and voice an opinion—even today, too many important software packages are written by programmers for programmers. Compatibility with other products is of course an important issue, and for many companies, integrated products which combine a word processor, spreadsheet, and database represent a cost-effective solution to a complex problem.

USER TRAINING

To enable employees to take the necessary responsibility for their welfare, and to minimize health risks, regulations require employers to provide their employees with information and training in the correct use of whatever computing they are expected to use. Normally this will mean, not a full-scale training course, but information and practical guidance to minimize risks: How to adjust equipment and furniture for personal comfort; how to achieve a healthy and relaxed posture; why and how to practice voluntary body movement; and when and why to take rest breaks.

The bottom line: Costs and benefits

The bottom line is that, sooner or later, all organizations will have to invest money in ergonomics. Non-compliant companies will be living on borrowed time. The good news is that compliance need not be expensive, and is undoubtedly good for you and your employees—and your company's productivity. It is also increasingly likely that many organizations will build compliance with current standards into their business contracts and purchase orders—if you don't comply, no one will buy. Remember, though, that the writers of the legislation are on the side of the corporations as well as the staff: It is in everyone's interest that companies should continue to thrive and grow even when legal constraints are imposed on them, so these guidelines provide ample leeway for companies to evaluate and respond cost-effectively to its requirements.

The cost of an audit is unavoidable, but independent auditors have the experience to recommend the most cost-effective solution and they have no product to sell, so if you are prepared and have a history of investment in staff comfort and personal development, you may be surprised at how little is actually required. Even modest investment in a comfortable working environment will yield the benefits of higher staff morale, productivity, and efficiency; a reduced risk of litigation, better staff retention, lower rates of absenteeism, and reduced health costs. Ergonomics is not a magic wand which will solve business problems, but it is a means of involving staff in the long-term future of the business and ensuring that they feel their well-being and their commitment are needed and valued. A compliant organization is one which will be set up, both legally and practically, to compete strongly in the marketplace and grow and develop within the framework of a safe and healthy environment—an attractive proposition for customers and employees alike.

Summary of tips for tackling office ergonomics

PREPARING TO TACKLE THE LEGISLATION

1. Think positive: Ergonomics is about improvements in productivity.
2. Don't look at the legislation as a frightening and expensive imposition on your business. It is simply a formalized extension of many good practices which are in use today and is designed to be simple and cheap to implement.
3. Don't impose changes: The legislation is supposed to enhance the working environment, not restrict it. You and your staff need to work as a team to ensure an optimum solution.
4. Appoint one person to take responsibility for the overall running and implementation of an ergonomics program. You don't need to have an in-house expert, just someone who may have an interest in the area or some experience in health and safety.
5. Find a concise summary of the current legislation to provide a framework for your strategy.
6. Productivity benefits greatly outweigh the costs of ergonomics. Compliance is an investment, not a penalty.
7. Apparent vagueness in current standards is an opportunity for you to define your own priorities and solutions: It is not a way for the law to catch you.

Environment

8. Don't be fooled by companies offering expensive, so-called "ergonomic accessories" which look interesting or attractive. Applying ergonomics successfully means standing back and studying the whole picture, and then applying a holistic solution.
9. A surprising amount can be achieved by persuading your staff to tidy up their office space. Tidily stacked boxes, clear walkways, and regularly filed paperwork will solve many of the "ergonomic" problems that offices are prone to.
10. Reorganize desks so that telephone and computer cables can't trip up passersby. Most office desks include slots or holes specifically for this purpose.
11. Avoid excessive contrast between lit and unlit areas. You will know if you are overlit (far more common than underlit) if your office includes areas of sharp shadow and excessive glare, or if your staff are prone to frequent headaches.
12. There are no generalizations which will satisfy all your staff. Ergonomics depends on the person, the situation, and the task.

Furniture

13. Try to choose chairs and desks together so that they complement one another. It is no use having the perfect chair if your desk is so low that it crushes your knees anyway.
14. Buy adjustable chairs, since no set of dimensions fits everyone. The height of the seat should be adjustable between 30 and 33 inches, and the backrest should tilt to support the user at work and at rest. Swivel chairs are preferable to stationary ones.
15. Chairs are most stable on a five-point base, which should include castors.
16. The controls of the chair should be easy to operate and within reach of the seated user—and make sure users know how they work!

17. Don't spend a fortune on so-called "ergonomic" chairs, many of which are little more than gimmicks. The backless knee-support chair, for example, puts excessive pressure on the knee and shin and doesn't always support the back.

18. Ergonomically engineered desks are expensive and should be restricted to people with a very specific need (designers, for instance, who need extra large or sloping tables, or those who are very tall or very short).

19. Standard office desks conform to height and depth criteria and are acceptable to most people. Supply footrests for smaller people and the option of an adjustable desk for tall people.

20. If two or more people are going to be using one work area, the equipment must be adjustable so that each can fit into his or her most comfortable working position.

COMPUTERS AND WORKSTATIONS

21. Angle monitors away from direct light sources to minimize glare. It is cheaper and frequently more effective than anti-glare screens.

22. Position monitors so that users look down at them at an angle of around 15 degrees. Maintain a distance of around 15 inches between face and screen to avoid eye strain.

23. Choose keyboards of three inch thickness (at the middle) with keys measuring somewhere between 1/4 -1/2 inches square. The angle of incline should be between 10 to 15 degrees. Keying action is often a matter of personal preference, but it is important that each depression should provide some form of feedback, such as a clicking noise or feel.

24. Keyboards must be detachable from the main computer. This goes without saying for desktop personal computers, but notebooks are a loophole. Don't let employees use notebooks as their main desktop machine—desirable as they are, they are not designed for prolonged use and will exacerbate musculoskeletal problems.

25. Don't over-react to emotional issues like radiation. There is no conclusive evidence that VDUs are harmful, and plenty of legislation is in place to control emission levels.

26. Be aware of other people's reactions to emotional issues like radiation. Although pregnant women are not legally entitled to insist on LCD screens, employers will gain by listening sympathetically to such requests.

PRINTERS, PERIPHERALS, AND ACCESSORIES

27. Put printers somewhere where they will not create noise pollution. Partitions or longer cables are usually enough to do the job.

28. If mice are widely used, make sure there is enough desk space for users to manipulate them without getting cramped. Of course, it is also the employees' responsibility to organize the desktop to accommodate a mouse.

29. System units, modems, and CD-ROM drives are cumbersome and work as well under as on the desk.

30. Document holders are important for copy typists. They also keep paper off the desk and out of the way.

SOFTWARE

31. Make sure you understand what users want to do before you buy the software to do it.

32. If you design your own software, test it on users as early and as frequently as possible.

33. Never underestimate the huge loss of productivity caused by badly designed, frustrating software. Too many users will not speak up because they blame themselves, so talk to manufacturers about the ways they try to get around this.

34. Don't take anyone's word for it when they claim their software is the easiest to use. Read usability reviews and ask for demonstrations or trial periods of the products you are considering.

35. Look for graphics, speech-like dialogue boxes, obvious Help, well designed manuals, and clear terminology.
36. Despite claims to the contrary, there is no software with which users will be fluent the first time. Expect some teething troubles, and be prepared to invest in training.
37. Don't feel obliged to buy all your applications from one manufacturer. If some users prefer one package and some another, it is in your interests to buy both, and it need not cause compatibility problems. If there is no strong feeling, however, go for consistency.
38. Think twice about buying obscure software from very small outlets. Support and clear future upgrade paths are always going to be important.

PEOPLE

39. Encourage a sense of personal responsibility in users for their working environment. Tidying a desk should be a therapeutic activity, not an enforced ritual.
40. Get users involved in buying decisions as soon as possible. Ergonomics is about physical comfort, so it helps to encourage physical testing of furniture, machinery, and software.
41. Steer clear of incentives which encourage more rapid data entry—all you will get is more errors, more RSI, and more litigation.
42. People care more when they have personal interests at stake: If employees are allowed to define their personal working space, they develop a sense of "ownership" and a greater feeling of responsibility.
43. Some people will be inseparable from a non-compliant chair or may refuse to wear protective clothing. Explain the legal position and if they still won't cooperate, get them to sign an affidavit relieving you of responsibility.
44. Don't panic! Everyone wins in a well-designed office.

Resources

Alexander, George. "Carpal Tunnel Syndrome and Other Cumulative Trauma Disorders" *The Seybold Report on Publishing Systems,* March 8, 1993, v22, n12, p12(9).

Arthur, Charles. "Keeping an Eye Out for Sonic the Hedgehog" *Newsbytes* March 4, 1993, pNEW03040007.

Becker, R. O. "The Link Between Electricity and Cancer" *Health Confidential,* January 1991, v5, n1.

Blakeslee, S. "Electromagnetic Fields Are Being Scrutinized for Linkage to Cancer" *The New York Times,* April 2, 1991.

Brodeur, Paul. "Annals of Radiation: The Hazards of Electromagnetic Fields III—Video Display Terminals" *Vanity Fair,* June 26, 1989.

Brody, Herb. "The Body in Question: How to Stay Healthy at the PC" *Newsbytes,* July 31, 1991, pNEW07310020.

Bulkeley, William. "Gender Affects How Users See Computers" *Wall Street Journal,* March 17, 1994.

Chandler, Doug. "Studies Provide Inconclusive Findings About Dangers of Monitor Emissions" *PC Magazine,* July 1991, v10, n13, p106(2).

Dvorak, John C. "The Servant Becomes the Master: The Computer Is Killing Us" *PC/Computing,* August 1993, v6, n8, p90(1).

Eabry, S. "The Invisible World of Electromagnetic Fields" *Parents' Press,* February 1991.

Flynn, Mary Kathleen. "Keyboards Split" *PC Magazine,* March 30, 1993, v12, n6, p31(1).

Flynn, Mary Kathleen. "Mice and Trackballs" *PC Magazine,* August 1990, v9, n14, p211(34).

Furger, Roberta. "Not For Your Eyes Only" *PC World,* February 1993, v11, n2, p34(1).

Gunn, Angela. "Healthier Typing With Keyboard Enhancements" *PC Magazine,* February 25, 1992, v11, n4, p314(2).

Haggett, Scott. "People Most Important When You're Changing Information Technology" *The Financial Post,* October 1991, p48(1).

Halliday, Caroline. "Monitor Vendors Address Flicker Issue" *PC/Computing,* March 1989, v2, n3, p140(6).

Hedge, Alan. "Bright Lights Blamed for Eye Fatigue" *The Edell Health Letter,* November 1990, v9,n10, p1(1).

Karon, Paul. "Making Humans Masters of Their Machines" *PC World,* February 1993, v11, n2, p34(1).

Kiesler, S. and T. Finholt. "The Mystery of RSI" *American Psychologist,* 1988, v43, n12, p1004-14.

Kotzsch, Ronald E. "Regain Grace: The Alexander Technique" *East West Natural Health,* March-April 1992, v22, n2, p38(3).

Louderback, Jim. "Notebook PCs Could Use a Little Usability Testing" *PC Week,* February 1, 1993, v10, n4, p60(1).

McCormick, John. "31 Unions Seek Anti-Repetitive Strain Injury Standards" *PC Week,* June 7, 1988, v5, n23, p144(2).

Mello, John P. Jr. "Keyboard Size: How Small is Too Small?" *Computer Shopper,* March 1993, v13, n3, p346(1).

Nadel, Brian. "The Green Machine" *PC Magazine,* May 25, 1993, v12, n10, p110(14).

Pereira, J. "Video Games Help Boys to Jump Onto Information Superhighway" *Wall Street Journal,* March 17, 1994.

Rosch, Winn L. "Does Your PC—Or How You Use It—Cause Health Problems?" *PC Magazine,* November 26, 1991, pp. 491-495.

Rosch, Winn L. "Monitor Emissions: Should Your Worry?" *PC Magazine,* December 12, 1989, v8, n21, p275(9).

Rosch, Winn L. "The Big Question: Is the PC Environment a Safe Place to Work?" *Cadcam,* March 1993, v12, n3, p25(4).

Rowell, Dave. "Is Your Monitor Safe?" *PC Week,* July 8, 1991, v8, n27, p105(2).

Rowinsky, Walt. "Quality of Monitor Affects Productivity, Comfort of Workers" *PC Week,* January 6, 1987, v4, n1, p99(3).

Seymour, Jim. "PC Ergonomics: Curing Office Ills" *Canadian Datasystems,* March 1990, v22, n3, p16(2).

Steinhart, Jim. "More Than Mere Frills: Computer Accessories" *PC Week,* November 26, 1990, v7, n47, p125(1).

White, R. *How Computers Work,* Ziff Davis Press, 1993.

Wilkes, Maurice. "Charles Babbage—The Great Uncle of Computing?" *Communications of the ACM,* March 1992, v35, n3, p15(3).

Wilmott, Don. "Carpal Tunnel Savior?" *PC Magazine,* March 30, 1993, v12, n6, p44(1).

Zucker, Paul. "Australia—Video Games Cleared in Epilepsy Scare" *Newsbytes,* February 17, 1993, pNEW02170003.

Index

D

E

F

G

H